Fast Lane to Fitness

The Busy Woman's Guide to Building A Sleek Physique In a Limited Amount of Time.

BY ROBERT KENNEDY AND DWAYNE HINES II

Published by MuscleMag International
6465 Airport Road
Mississauga, ON
Canada L4V 1E4

Designed by Jackie Kydyk
Edited by Mandy Morgan

10 9 8 7 6 5 4 3 2 1 Pbk.

Canadian Cataloguing In Publication Data

Kennedy, Robert, 1938-
Fast lane to fitness: the busy woman's guide to building a
sleek physique in a limited amount of time

Includes index.
ISBN 1-55210-012-X

1.Physical fitness for women. I.Hines, Dwayne, 1961-
II.Title.

RA781.6.K35 1998 613.7'045 C98-900958-0

Distributed in Canada by
CANBOOK Distribution Services
1220 Nicholson Road
Newmarket, ON
L3Y 7V1
800-399-6858

Distributed in the States by
BookWorld Services
1933 Whitfield Park Loop
Sarasota, FL 34243
800-444-2524

Printed in Canada

Warning

This book is not intended as medical advice, nor is it offered for use in the diagnosis of any health condition or as a substitute for medical treatment and/or counsel. Its purpose is to explore advanced topics on sports nutrition and exercise. All data are for information only. Use of any of the programs within this book is at the sole risk and choice of the reader.

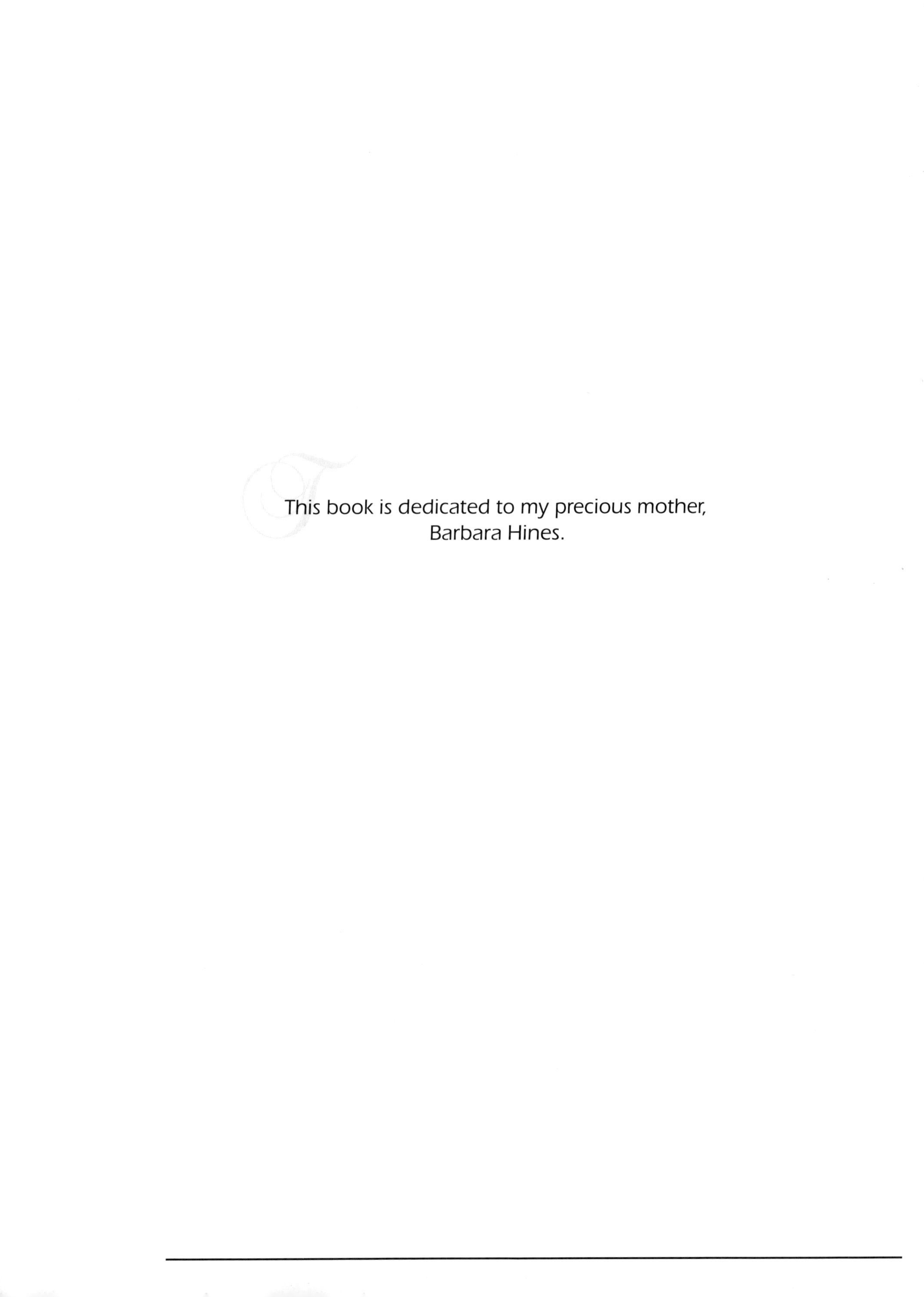

This book is dedicated to my precious mother,
Barbara Hines.

Table of Contents

Can A Busy Woman Really Get Into Shape?

Every year millions of people make New Year's resolutions – plans and goals for changing their life for the better. One of the major areas of concern, and often the most dwelled upon resolution pertains to the body. People really want to increase their level of health and fitness. They want to lose 20 pounds of fat, gain some muscularity, lose a couple of inches off of their waist, or tighten their legs and arms. People care about how they look, and how they feel. They care about their health. Most people want to do more than just survive, they want to thrive. Living well encompasses many things and one central aspect is physical health. Fitness plays an important role in "better" living according to most peoples' definitions. It really doesn't matter how much money you have if your body is not up to par.

The desire for a fit and healthy physique often clashes with the realities of life. For example, most people start the year with a variety of ideas about getting into shape, yet fail any attempts to actualize their goals. The gyms and health clubs that were overloaded for the first couple of weeks in January soon dwindle back to their pre-New Year membership size. The fitness equipment many people bought soon sits idle, collecting dust in the corner. The desired goals for most people remain just that – unrealized desires, not attainments. They never seem to get a handle on how to handle their physiques. These problems are especially true for the busy women tackling today's world.

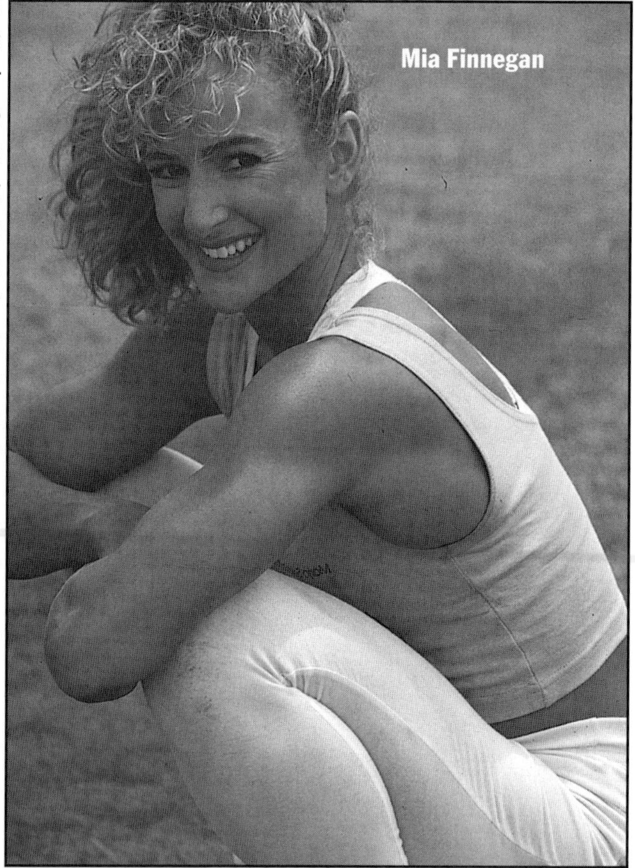
Mia Finnegan

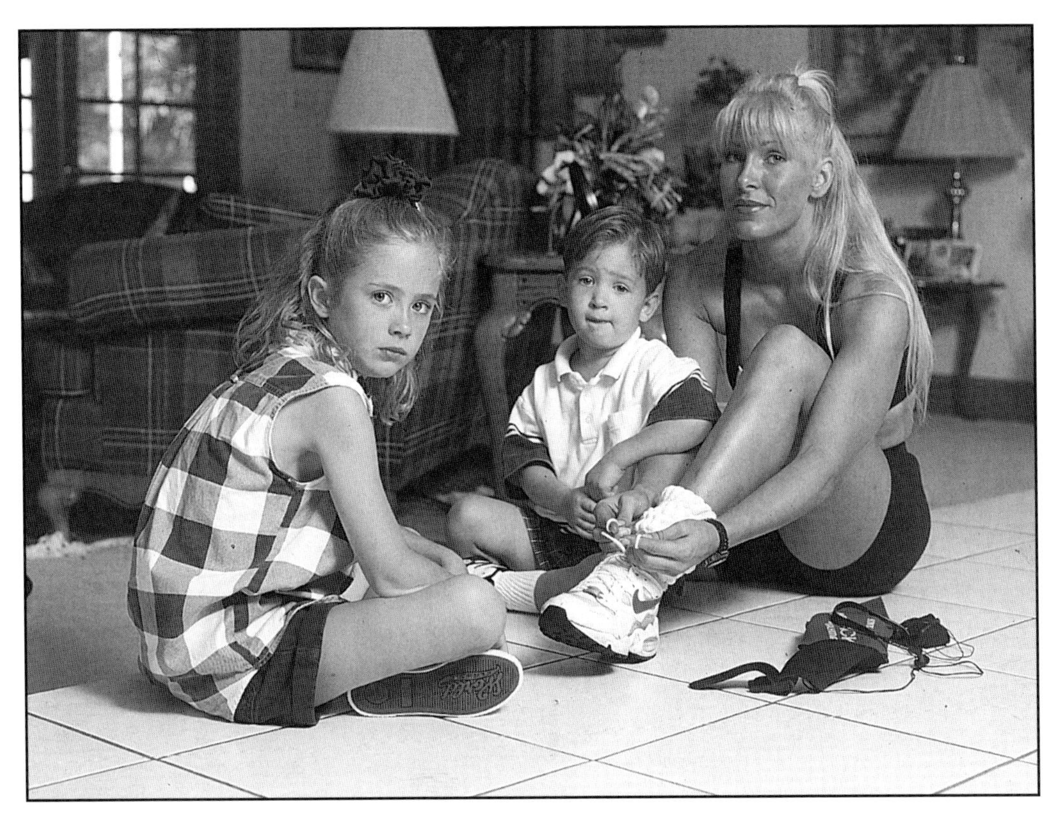

Time

One of the major obstacles standing in the way of a great physique is time – or lack of it. There is simply not enough time to do everything you need or want to get done. Husband, children, work, extended family, outside activities, group meetings, holidays, and dozens of other commitments and obligations add up to make short work of your week. As you grow older you seem to accumulate more and more responsibilities which take up even more time out of your overloaded week. One of the areas that gets squeezed out of your weekly activities is the care of your physique. Your body often ends up with the short straw. In the mad swirl to get everything done you tend to overlook the needs of your physique. This is unfortunate because your body has certain needs which should not go neglected. These aspects concern health, fitness, and appearance. Neglecting these areas leads to an unbalanced lifestyle, which cuts into all areas of your life. That is, if you neglect your body to focus on other areas, the other areas will also suffer in the long run due to the eventual demise of the physique. When you do not pay sufficient attention to your body it will not function at its full potential in any area.

If you neglect your body to focus on other areas of your life, these areas will also eventually suffer as your health fails.

FAST FITNESS GUIDANCE

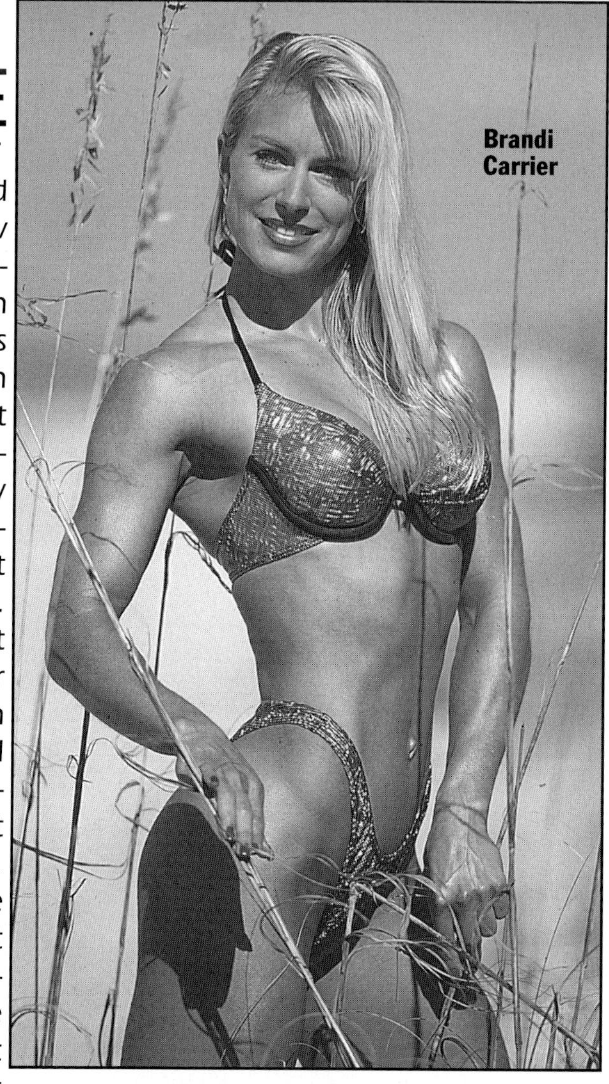

Most people know they need to exercise more. They also know they need to pay special attention to their diet. What has been general common knowledge is now official – the Surgeon General has determined that lack of physical activity is detrimental to your health. So now everyone knows what was suspected all along – you can't get away with being out of shape. However, this knowledge (that you need to work on your body, but don't have enough time to do so) just seems to add more stress to daily living. Knowing you need fitness, but not being able to do much about it, doesn't help either. That's where *Fast Lane to Fitness* comes in. It is possible to make some significant changes to your physique in short periods of time. Just because you do not have a lot of time for fitness does not mean you have to totally neglect your body. The key to successful fitness is consistency, not necessarily long workouts. In fact, some people actually set their physiques back by training too much.

The Surgeon General has determined that lack of physical activity is detrimental to your overall health.

You can build a fit and healthy body even if you only have a limited amount of time available.

Consistency and persistence are the essential elements of a good fitness program, and they can be applied to shorter workout schedules as well. Consistency is a powerful tool for controlling the body. A consistent workout program and a consistently solid, nutritious diet can conquer the body. Even if you don't have a lot of time to spare, working on your physique consistently can make a big difference. Fitness star Tatiana Anderson relates in *Muscle Media 2000* (September 1995) that "consistency is very important. You have to make it a habit."

The good news is that it is possible to get into great shape even when you only have a limited amount of time to do so. The key is to know what to do, how to do it, and then organize a quick, cohesive routine. Most people miss out on this point, but not to worry, *Fast Lane to Fitness* contains the guidelines needed for how and what you need to do, and it is organized for you. All you need to do to get into shape is to follow the guidelines outlined in *Fast Lane to Fitness* on a consistent basis. They are directed toward the women who only have a limited amount of time available for building a sleek and healthy physique.

Consistency conquers the physique.

COMMITMENT AND CONSISTENCY

The primary elements you can use to get your body into shape are commitment and consistency. The time element (lack of enough time) can be beaten if you have these two factors working for you. A strong commitment to fitness will keep you at the task of controlling your physique, and consistency provides the base from which the body can grow. Hit-and-miss training is not very effective for shaping your physique. On the other hand, a consistent weekly fitness pattern, even if it is brief, is effective. Again, consistency is more important than length when it comes to fitness. Consistency and commitment are the major pillars of success in almost any endeavor, especially when it comes to training the physique.

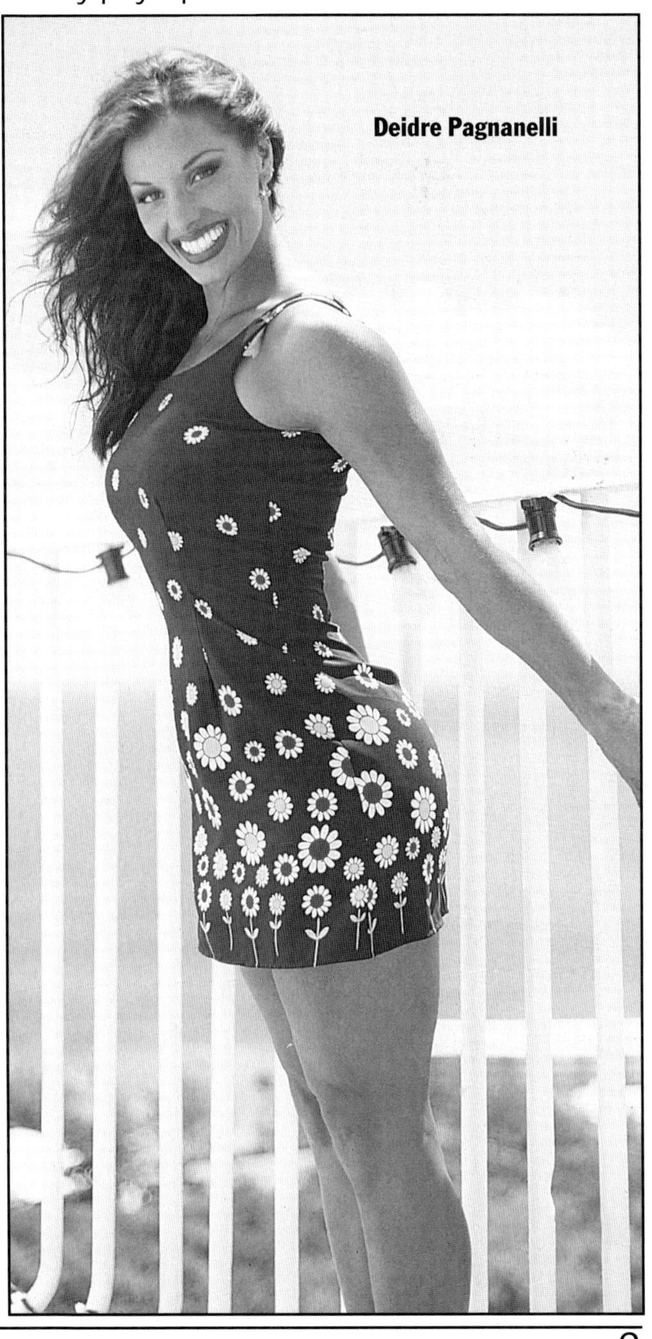
Deidre Pagnanelli

Your will power can be amazingly strong – direct it at improving your physique.

The quickest way to positively change your physique is to increase muscularity while decreasing bodyfat levels.

Commitment and consistency are inner qualities – personal characteristics that can be cultivated through personal discipline. The main driving force in stirring up consistency and commitment is your will – you have to "want" to achieve your goals, to passionately go after them. Fitness star Mia Finnegan is someone who has amazing will power; it has paid off for her – just look at her beautiful physique. The women who have consistently done well in fitness competitions, such as Debbie Kruck, Monica Brant, Carol Semple-Marzetta and Brandi Carrier, etc., are people who have been consistent and committed. You have to strongly desire change. You have to build and maintain motivation for the process of changing your physique. It is a part of self-discipline. You use self-discipline in other areas of your life such as raising your children and taking care of the responsibilities at work. Now simply apply the same discipline to your physique and you can make significant gains there as well. Your will is very powerful, an "inner" muscle, so to speak, of immense strength. When you completely focus it on an area in your life, you can move mountains. Direct your will power towards improving your physique on a consistent basis and you can build a better body.

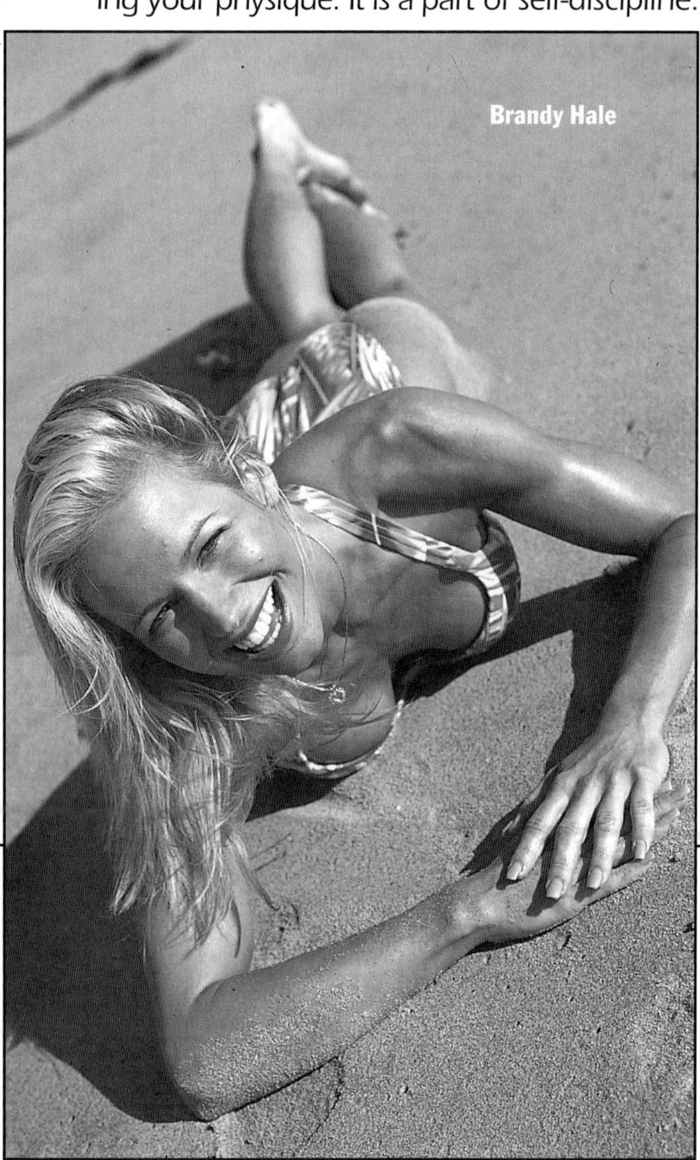
Brandy Hale

BUILDING A BETTER BODY

The goal of the *Fast Lane to Fitness* program is to get you into good condition under the constraint of time. Getting into good condition means improving your health, fitness, and appearance. There are a few physical attributes that can be noticeably improved. These include your strength, endurance, and flexibility. In parallel, your appearance will also change, becoming leaner, trimmer, and more muscular. You will add muscle tone in some areas (such as the chest, shoulders, arms, etc.) while losing fat in other areas (such as the waist, hips, and even the chin). Increasing muscle tone and losing bodyfat is a dynamic combination. If you just lost fat without adding noticeable muscle tone, or increased muscle tone without losing fat, the physical change would be less apparent, as would the health benefits. But when both occur, you take notice of the positive changes much quicker. As you will see, *Fast Lane to Fitness* works on both areas – losing fat and increasing muscle tone, which promotes an increase in your health, fitness, and appearance.

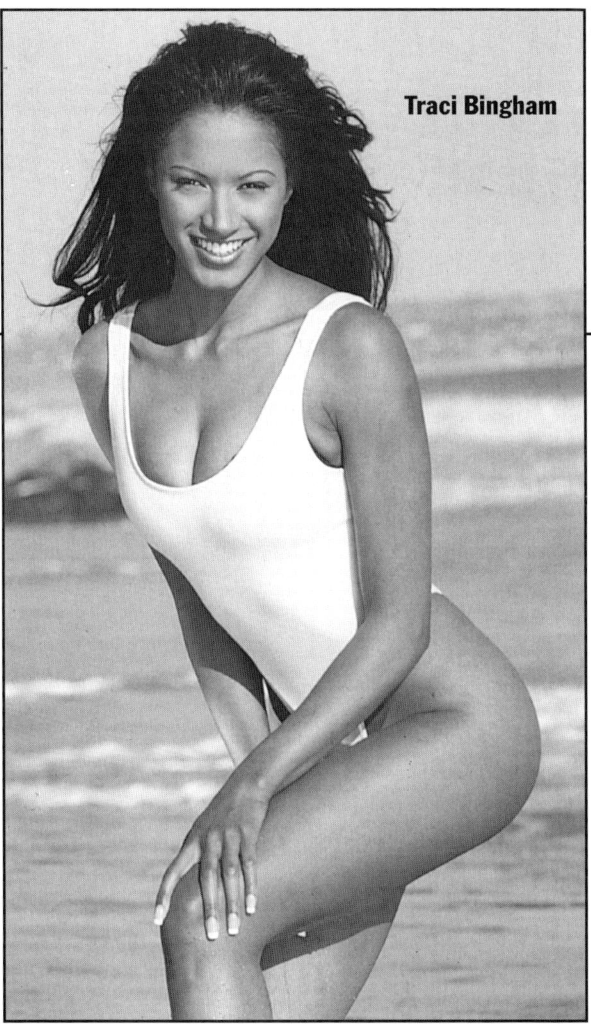
Traci Bingham

UNIVERSAL APPLICATION

The principles and guidelines contained in *Fast Lane to Fitness* have a universal application – they work for both men and women. Since this book is written for women, the spotlight will be on a woman's body training and conditioning needs. Some women may be concerned about becoming too "muscular" if they work out with physique shaping tools such as weights. In general, this fear is unfounded. *Muscle & Fitness* magazine (November 1996) notes that "when a woman trains like a man, won't she end up looking like a man? – No, but if she trains right, she will develop stronger muscles and a shapelier body." Women do not have the testosterone levels that men have and do not need to worry about becoming too "bulked up." The sports women who do get larger are often taking drugs to do so. If you train naturally you won't have to worry about this problem. Michelle Basta Boubion points out in *Muscle & Fitness* (November 1996) that training will do a lot for a woman: increase her metabolic rate (which helps burn off fat throughout the day), increase her muscle tone (which will

***Fast Lane to Fitness* works well for both men and women who need to get in shape but only have a limited amount of time available.**

act as a preventative against injuries and drastically improves the appearance), increase her shapeliness, and increase bone density, which is particularly beneficial for the female physique.

Training will also increase health levels and self-image. People sometimes overlook the significance body conditioning can have on personal confidence, but it should not be overlooked because it can be very beneficial. Training also promotes a significantly shapelier body in overall appearance. Nancy Georges, winner of the Ms. Fitness USA title, related in an *Ironman* article (September 1994) that she once was very thin, thin to the point that she would be made fun of. Therefore she took up training, combining weights and aerobic work, transforming her physique from lanky, to shapely. Nancy's muscular curves have won fitness physique competitions for her on a national level. Sharon Bruneau came from a modeling and dancing background, and found that fitness training, particularly using weights, helped her to really improve her shape and appearance. These are not isolated incidents. Women find that fitness training, including weight training, is excellent for shaping their physiques as well as benefiting their overall health. Physique star and model Marjo Selin notes in *MuscleMag International* that "bodybuilding women are strong and beautiful. We have no limits."

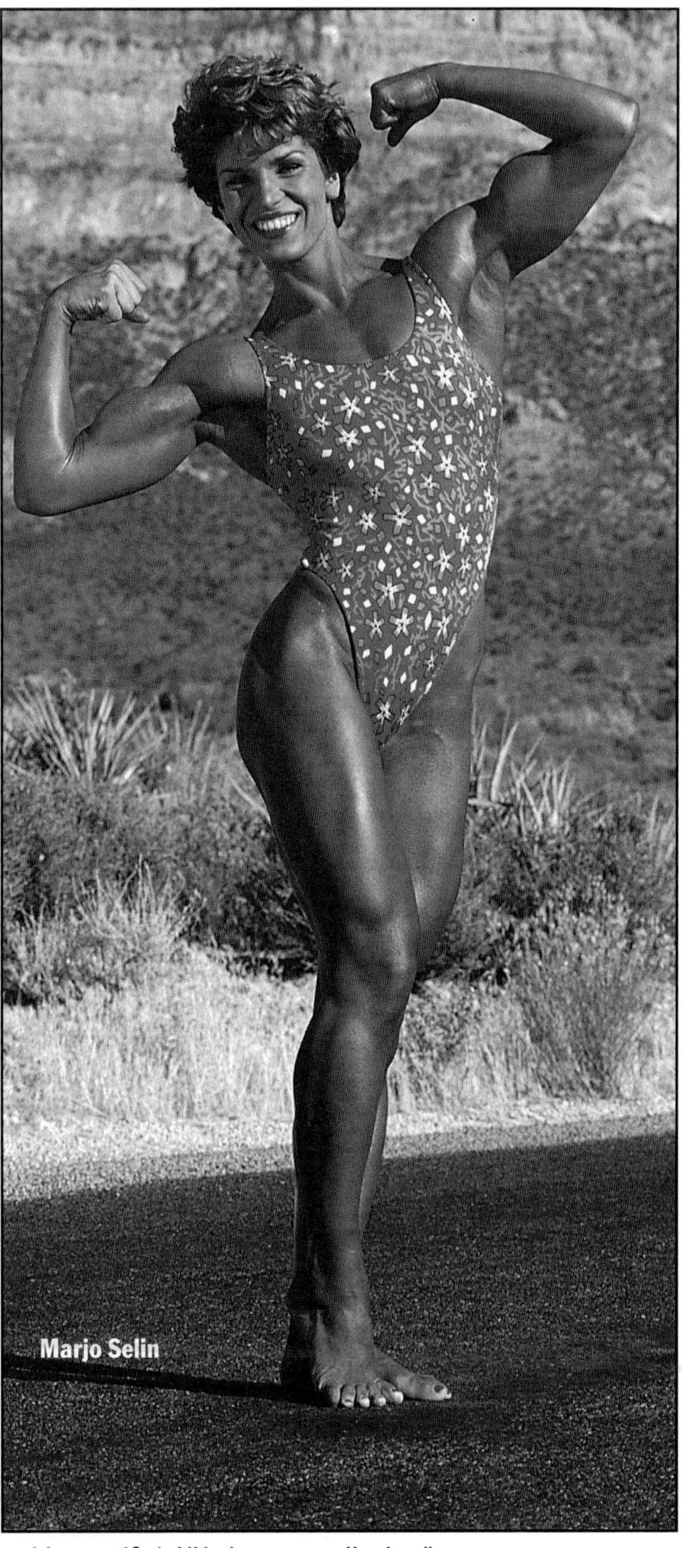
Marjo Selin

Fast Lane to Fitness, which is based on the best fitness principles, works well for the woman who is busy but still wants to get into great shape.

Women have different goals in their personal pursuit of fitness, but the primary fitness principles in *Fast Lane to Fitness* can be used effectively to achieve those varied goals, whatever they are. Use the program, tailor it to your needs, and make the changes you want to your body.

ORGANIZED APPROACH

Do you let your children make chaos out of your home? Do you work in chaos? Do you or your husband turn in work assignments when you feel like it? Do you make a meal by just guessing at the ingredients? No, not if you want things to turn out right. You use an organized approach in the various areas of life. You use a time line and schedules. Work flows well when you are organized. The same holds true for fitness training. If you use a chaotic approach to getting in shape you will get little or no results. One of the major reasons why some women's fitness programs fail (in addition to lack of time) is lack of an organized training approach. Many people don't know what they are doing when it comes to fitness. They approach it in a chaotic manner, mixing a little of this with a little of that, making a mess. For fitness to be successful it needs to be organized into a unified approach. That is how things work in the real world and it is how things work with your physique. Most people don't have all of the pieces of the fitness puzzle, let alone know how to link them together in the proper manner. Even top athletes make mistakes when it comes to bringing all of the aspects of fitness together. For instance, the man considered "the world's fittest man," Ironman Mark

Successful fitness is organized fitness.

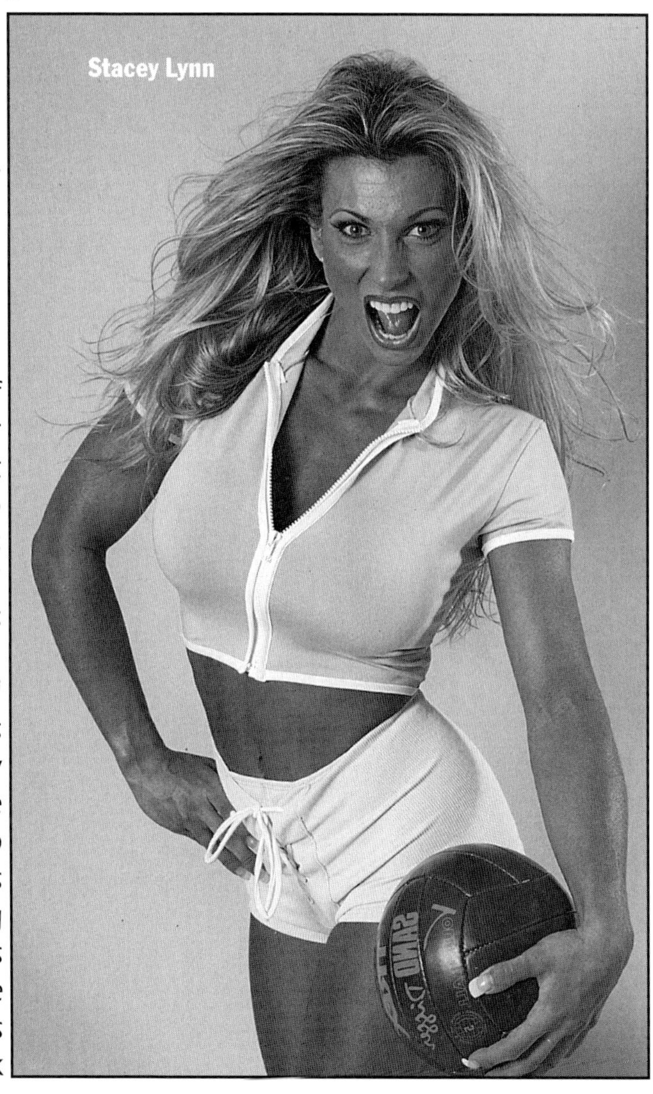
Stacey Lynn

Many people are confused when it comes to fitness. *Fast Lane to Fitness* provides a clear and concise approach to getting into top shape.

Allen, found himself floundering when he started using weights. He would go to the gym, mess around with a few dumbells, and leave without any inkling of what he'd actually done or exactly why he'd done it. "I remember looking around the gym and thinking, 'If I'm Mr. Ironman, supposedly the fittest guy in the world, and I don't know what I'm doing in here, then 95 percent of the other people don't either' " (*Outside*, February 1997). This confusion about how and what to do is a common occurrence for many people. That is why *Fast Lane to Fitness* will give you an edge. *Fast Lane to Fitness* brings the various streams of fitness (such as aerobic work, flexibility, and strength training) into one large river of concentrated activity, which will reshape your body into a sharper, healthier, and fitter you! What makes *Fast Lane to Fitness* so appropriate for the busy woman is that the various fitness elements are condensed to fit into any schedule. Not only are the various elements of fitness brought together into one group, but they are also condensed to a point where women on the go can still benefit from them. The *Fast Lane to Fitness* program brings together the essentials, necessary to shape the physique, and packages them into a brief format that works great even in the midst of a busy schedule. You do not have to spend time exploring and finding out about all of the intricacies of shaping your physique. You can use the guidelines provided in this book as a shortcut to what would have taken years to find out.

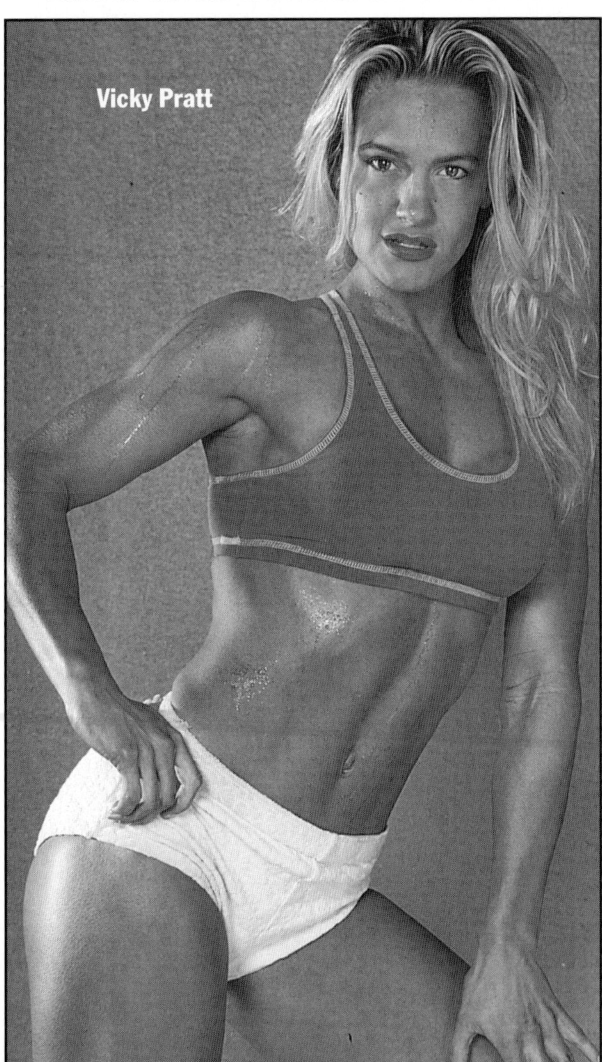
Vicky Pratt

Reading this book will let you know what to do, but it won't shape your body for you. You have to apply the principles and techniques to attain the physique you desire.

Good fitness has many aspects, and each needs to be addressed.

TOTAL BODY TRAINING

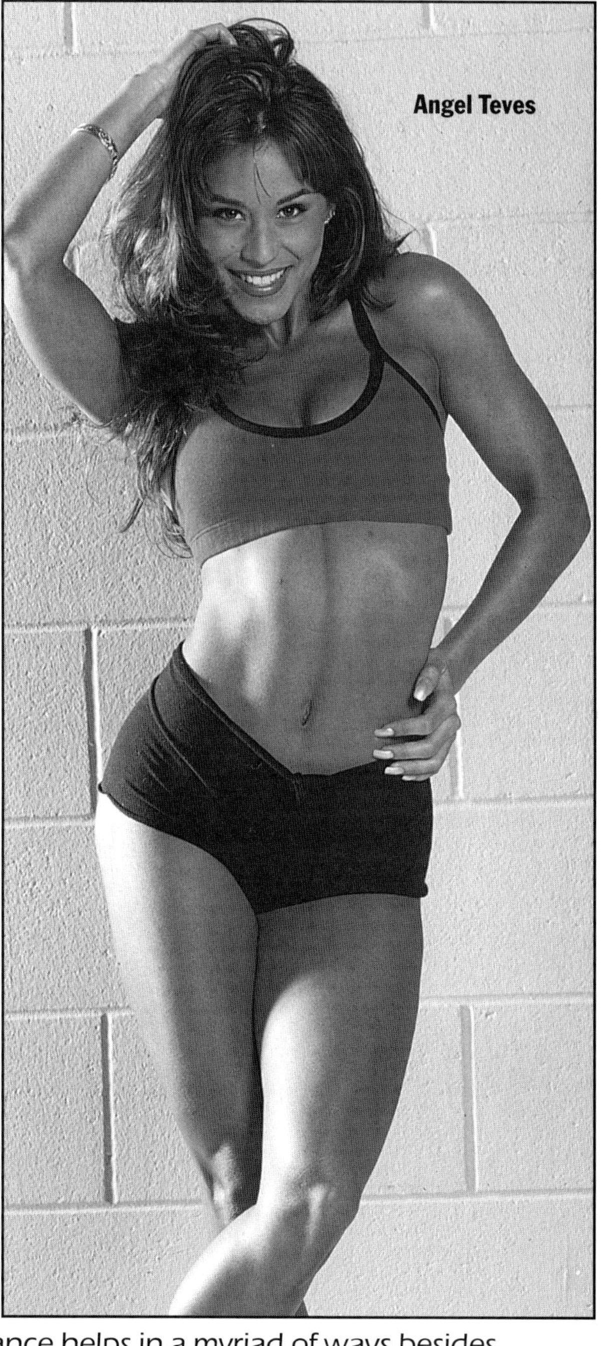
Angel Teves

There are numerous elements that make up the arena entitled fitness; *Fast Lane to Fitness* focuses on these areas most important to the overall fitness package. You cannot expect to take charge of your body by only hitting one area. For instance, you might go on a diet to lose some weight, but find that your body is still not as tight as you want it. This is because you also need to build your muscles, in addition to losing fat. Good fitness has many aspects, and each needs to be addressed. Upcoming chapters in *Fast Lane to Fitness* will be devoted to areas such as endurance training, strength and shape training, and flexibility.

Total fitness is addressed by bringing all of the elements of fitness into one schedule. Chapter five does this, integrating the physical activities into one group of weekly training sessions, condensed for the busy woman.

BENEFITS

The benefits of a good fitness program are vast. It is common knowledge that a fit and healthy lifestyle can help you live longer. A healthy lifestyle also helps you enjoy the years that you do live that much more. A sharper appearance helps in a myriad of ways besides just health, as it boosts your personal stock in relational, social, and business arenas. Looking great is not the only factor in success, but it certainly provides a strong hand. Additionally, healthy employees are absent from work less, and tend to both contribute more and make more money. People often work hard all of their lives only to end up unable to enjoy the fruits of their labor due to poor health. Paying attention to your health and fitness now will help you enjoy more of life later on. Fitness is not something you try to add to your retirement years alone – you should be working on fitness

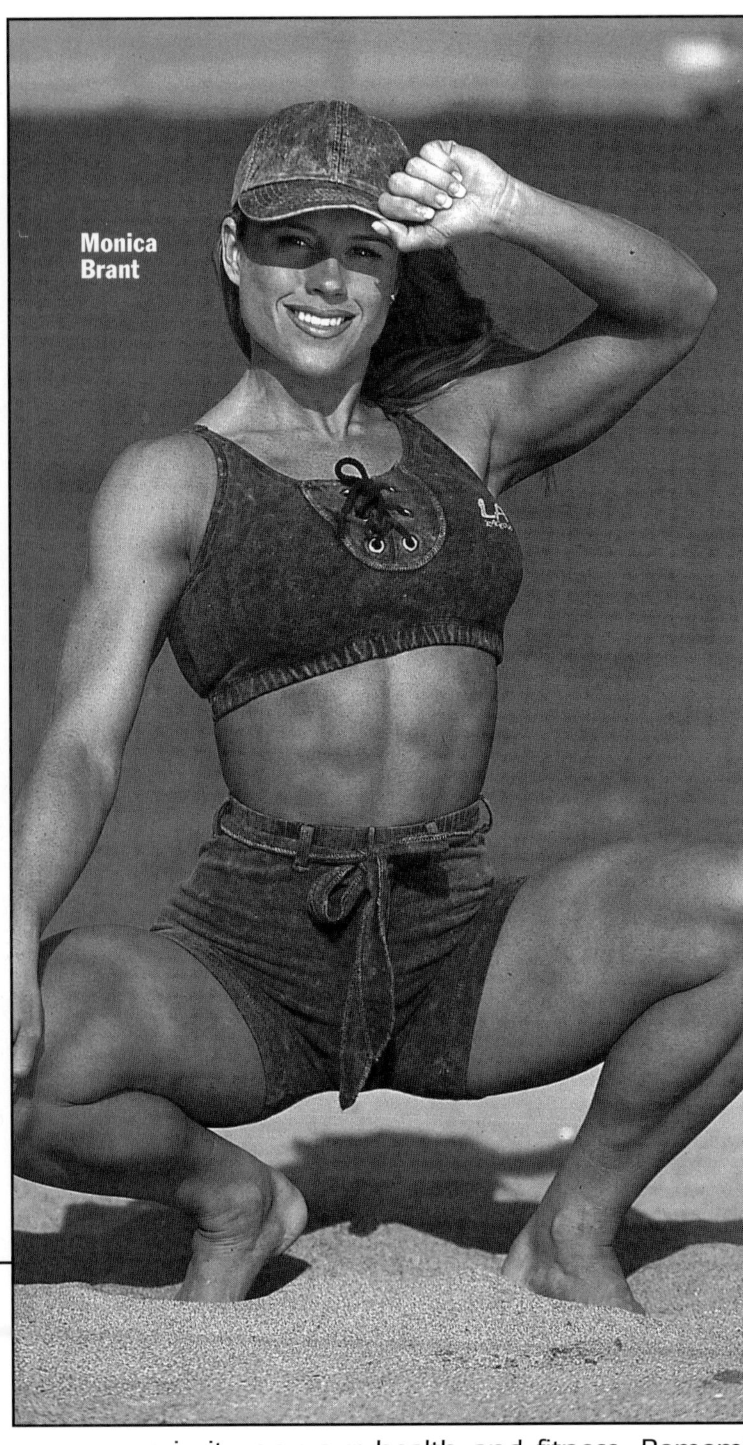

Monica Brant

throughout your life. *Fast Lane to Fitness* presents an approach to achieving a healthy lifestyle, no matter how hectic your life may seem.

Regular exercise elevates your mood on a regular basis, helping you to handle the daily stresses of life.

Yet another benefit of the fitness lifestyle is the reduction of stress. Most people face a number of different stressors throughout the day. When a person is always on the go, under deadlines, pressures, and responsibilities, stress can take a toll. An active lifestyle is a great way to reduce stress. Regular exercise elevates your mood on a regular basis, helping you handle the daily stresses of life.

PRIORITY

People tend to make room in their weekly schedules for the things they consider most important. Place a priority on your health and fitness. Remember, this does not mean an enormous time commitment. But it does mean a minimal amount of time carved out of your busy schedule on a weekly basis. The upcoming chapters provide specific guidance on getting in a brief but effective weekly workout, which will help transform the appearance of your physique. Even if you have a busy schedule there is still hope for your health and fitness through the use of the *Fast Lane to Fitness* training approach.

Start with a workout that gets you into the groove of things, and then gradually work into a more challenging workout routine.

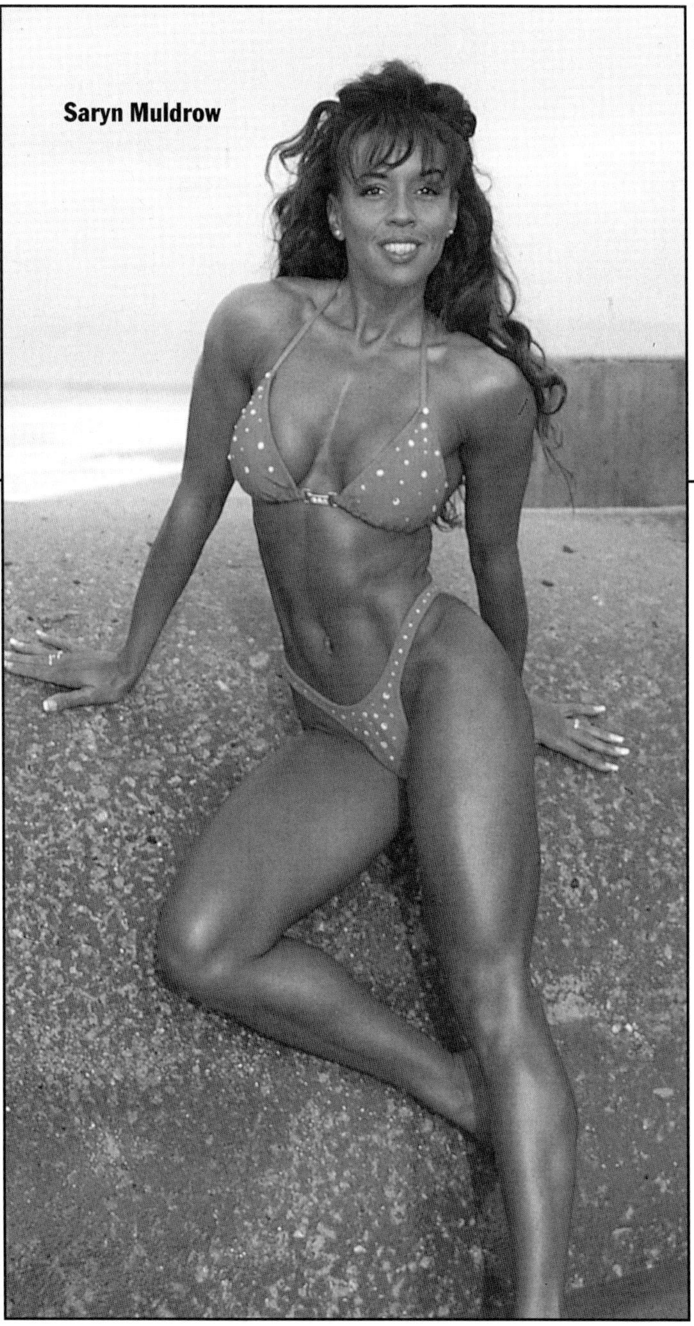

The first step is to get your doctor's approval before you start working out. Some people may have conditions that necessitate a slower move into fitness training. However, most likely, your doctor will give you the green light. Doctors tend to encourage people to get into fitness to promote better living. Get the blessing of your doctor, particularly if you are over 30 years of age and have never trained before or have not trained in the recent past.

Saryn Muldrow

GRADUAL PROGRESSION

Start slow as you begin your fitness routine. Rome wasn't built in a day and a great physique doesn't happen overnight. One of the primary keys to successfully transforming your physique is gradual progression. Don't try to do everything at once. You'll only end up overloading your body and burning it out right away. Let your body gradually become accustomed to the challenge of fitness. The best approach is to crawl before you walk. Start with a workout that gets you into the groove of things, and then gradually work into a more challenging workout routine. The routines mentioned in *Fast Lane to Fitness* should all be performed at your

Place a priority on your health and fitness.

A fit and healthy lifestyle provides a vast amount of personal benefits.

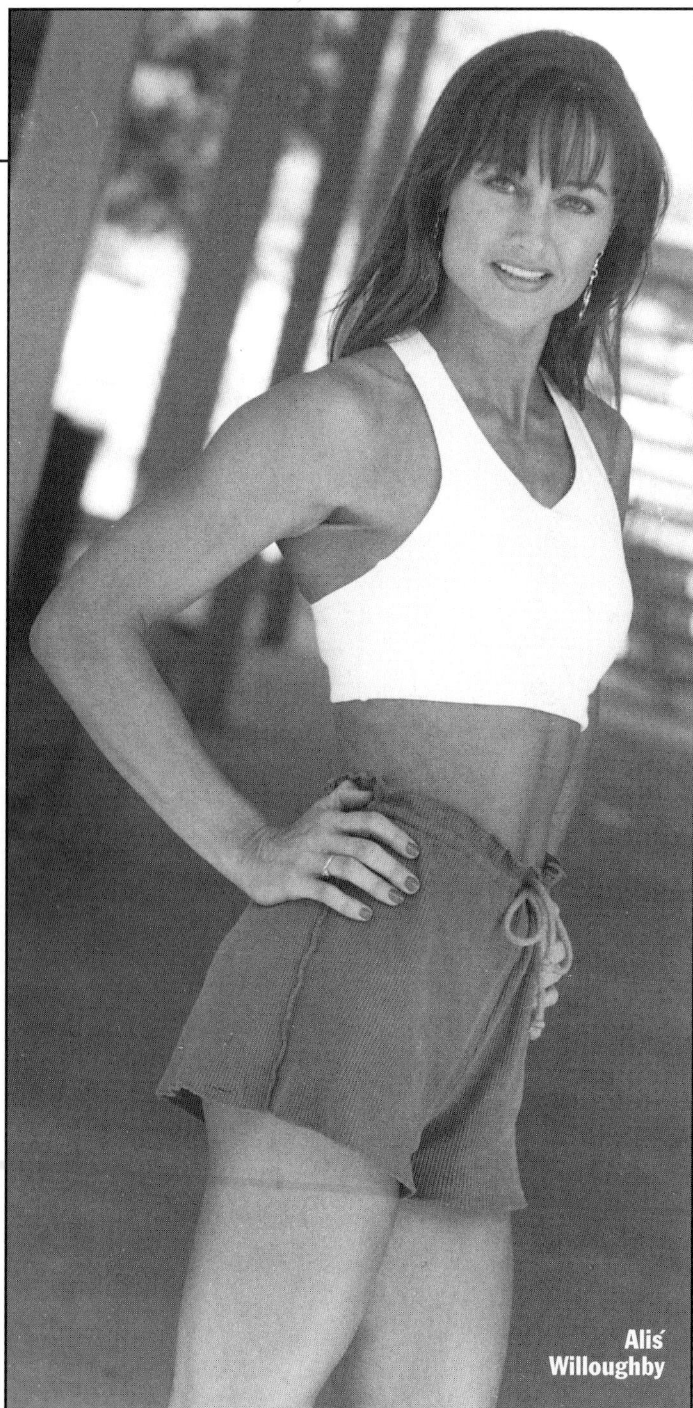
Alis´ Willoughby

present level of fitness. Once you have a few weeks of working out behind you, you can gradually increase the intensity of your workout.

ONE WEEK AT A TIME

You can get into shape, even if you have a busy schedule. The key is to use the guidance in this book to get in a few brief workouts a week on a consistent basis. Gradually work into the *Fast Lane to Fitness* program. Don't try and do everything at once. Focus on making the most of each week, and over time you will begin to see some impressive changes in your physique. Devote your total mental and physical assets to your workout when you do have the opportunity to get one in. The more focused and intense you become, the more progress you will see.

Use this book as your guide for getting into shape in an organized, progressive manner. Get into the *Fast Lane to Fitness* and start to take control of your body, even if you only have a brief amount of time to do so. The benefits are more than worth the effort. A sleek, streamlined body is not out of reach – it can be yours with the right mental outlook and proper training program.

Consistently follow the guidelines in this book to build the body you desire.

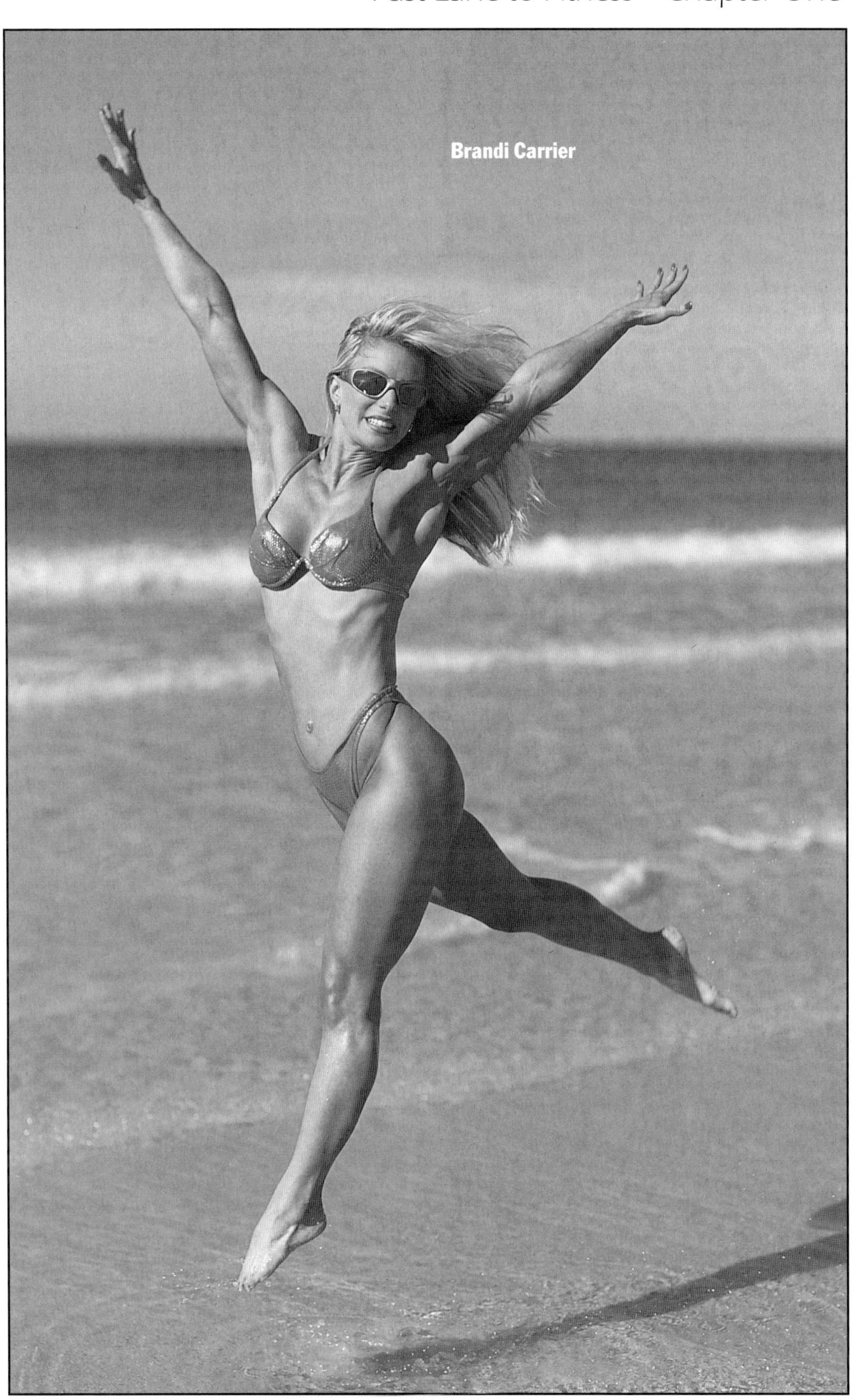
Brandi Carrier

Endurance and the Cardio Connection

There are several central aspects involved in training the physique and one of the most prominent is endurance training. Endurance training is training that extends over a period of time, and which builds up the body's endurance capacities. Endurance training is quite different from strength training. Strength training is more brief in nature than endurance training. Endurance training is aerobic in nature whereas strength training is anaerobic. The definition of aerobic means "with oxygen."

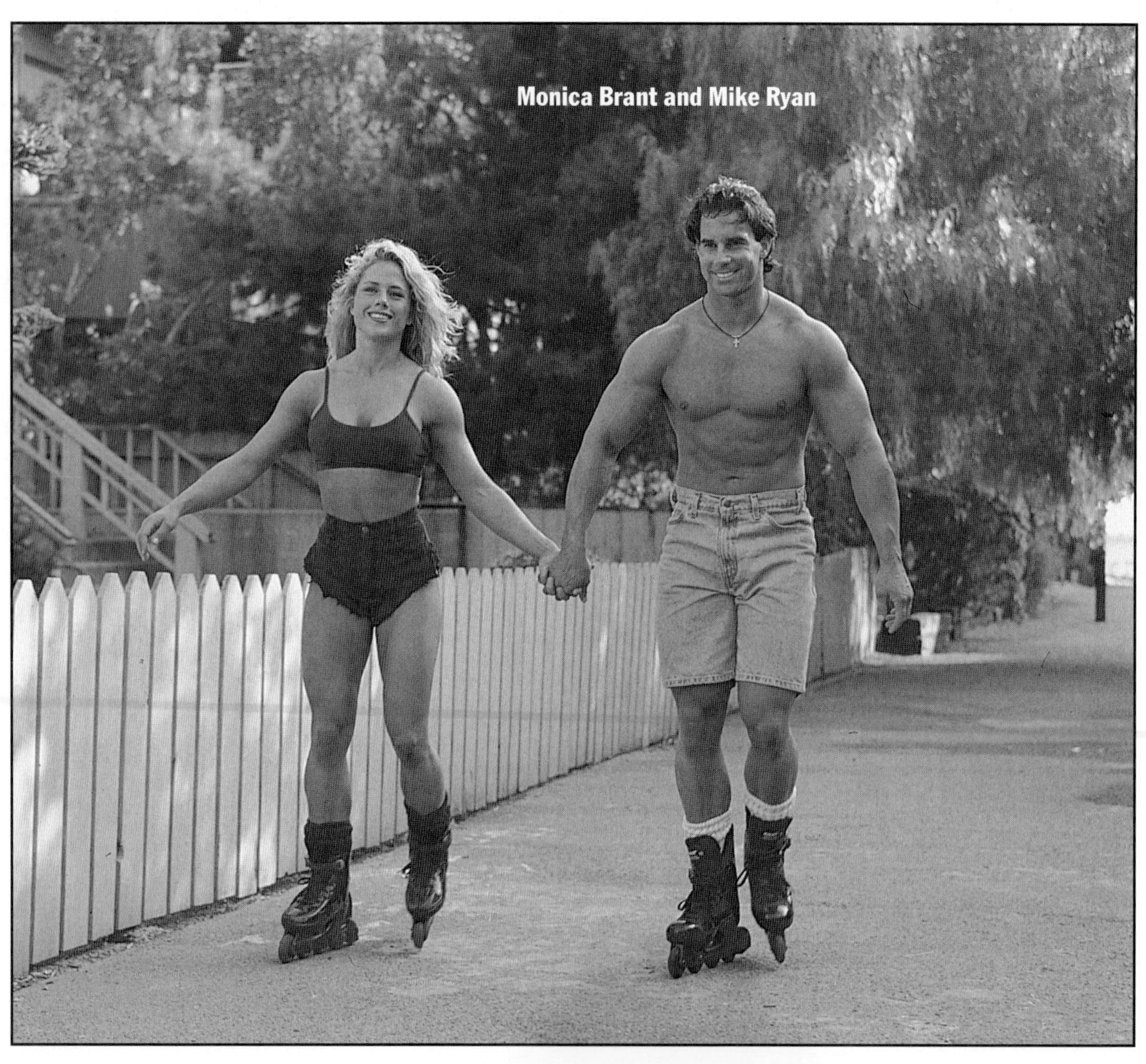

Monica Brant and Mike Ryan

An article in *Muscle & Fitness* (January 1996) on aerobics points out:

If you can only perform one type of exercise, choose aerobic exercise since it is so vital to your health.

In aerobic exercise, oxygen is involved in the metabolic processes that produce energy. Anaerobic exercise, on the other hand, depends upon energy produced in the absence of oxygen. Anaerobic exercise involves short bursts of intense effort, and is fueled by ATP stored in the muscles (which lasts only a few seconds) and glycogen. Aerobic exercise can be maintained for much longer periods than anaerobic work, although at a much lower level of intensity. Aerobic-energy metabolism draws on both glycogen and fat. In general, aerobic activity involves effort at a low level of intensity which can be maintained for long periods. The longer you continue this type of activity, the greater proportion of fat you use as fuel.

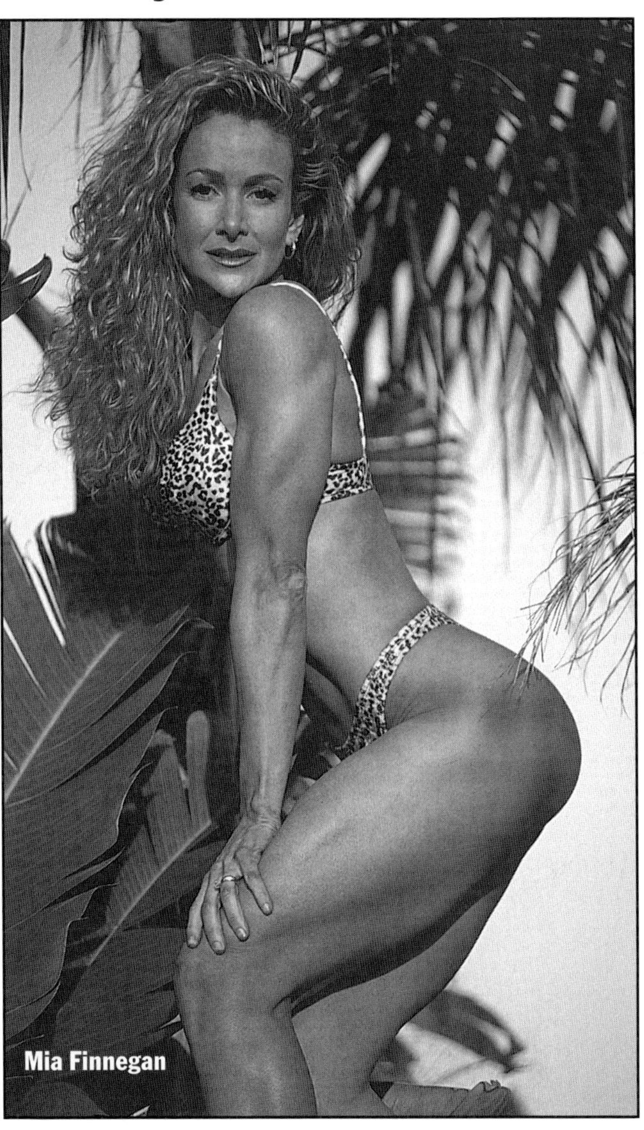
Mia Finnegan

Aerobic training is endurance training, the type of training performed at a low level of intensity (as compared to the high-level intensity of strength exercises), lasting for a long period of time. This type of training uses some glycogen (primarily in the initial stages of the workout), but mostly fat for fuel. This means that aerobic workouts are going to burn off bodyfat. Fitness stars such as Monica Brant, Mia Finnegan and others incorpoate aerobic workouts into their training programs. They recognize that aerobic training is essential for burning off bodyfat.

Another term for aerobic exercise is cardiovascular exercise. Cardiovascular exercise really gets the heart and lungs involved in a major manner (hence the name) and also involves raising the heart rate to a certain range. It has been noted (*Muscle & Fitness*, January 1996) that of all the fitness components (strength training, flexibility, etc.) cardiovascular endurance impacts health, disease resistance, and longevity the most. This translates into the important point that if you can only perform one aspect of a fitness program, make it the cardiovascular aspect. When the Surgeon General determined that lack of physical activity is detrimental to health, one of the most basic issues dealt with was cardiovascular health. If your cardiovascular health goes, you are in real trouble. So make cardiovascular fitness an essential part of your weekly schedule.

Cardiovascular exercise and aerobic exercise are one and the same, and most people use the terms interchangeably. In fact, good cardio exercise is aerobic in nature, and good aerobic exercise is cardiovascular in nature. The term cardio/aerobic exercise is often used, but we will use aerobic exercise in *Fast Lane to Fitness* to define the type of endurance training that works the heart and lungs at the proper intensity and which also burns off fat – long, low-intensity continuous exercise involving the major muscle groups. Since this type of exercise is so vital to overall fitness and health (the premium exercise), it is the first exercise focused upon in *Fast Lane to Fitness.*

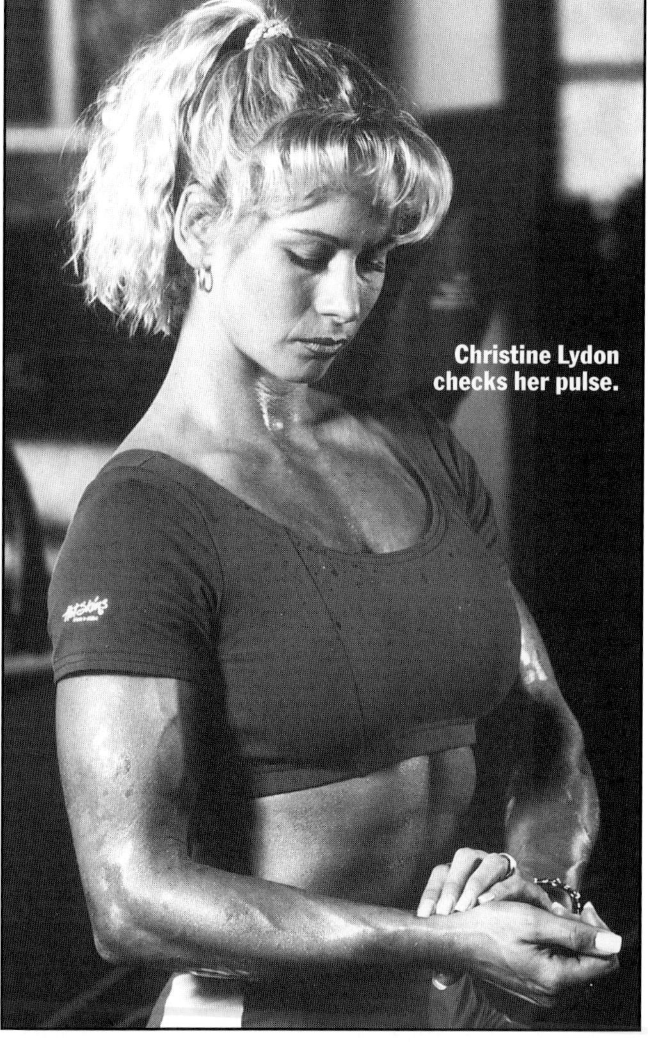

Christine Lydon checks her pulse.

TARGET HEART RATE

With aerobic exercise, it is important to work out in your target heart-rate range. This is the rate at which you are working hard enough to get your heart to a certain percentage of your maximum heart rate (MHR). Your maximum heart rate is determined by your age. Subtract your age from the number 220, then multiply the remainder by 60 percent and 85 percent (0.6 and 0.85). The lower number is the pulse beats per minute you should aim for when starting an aerobic program; the higher number is the beats per minute you aim for after you've trained a few months and are in shape. Exercise heart rates of 70 to 75 percent are also effective if you feel more comfortable at these levels. Use common sense in adjusting your intensity levels.[1]

Using common sense when adjusting your target heart-rate levels comes easy once you have been working out for a while, but what about when you are just getting started?

Start out by keeping your heart rate around 60 to 65 percent of your maximum (above 50 percent might be a good starting level for some people). As you build stamina, aim for 70 to 75 percent. Don't push so hard that you feel dizzy, faint, or nauseated, or can't continue for 30 minutes. If the work seems easy, push harder by moving faster or increase the incline or the level if on a machine.[2]

It should be noted that the 30-minute range is for those who have worked up to that range; you do not necessarily want to start off with a 30-minute workout, particularly if you are just getting into the fitness scene (the length of your aerobic workout will be discussed in the upcoming pages).

A table is provided for you to get a good estimate of the target heart rate you want to work out at. To get a good idea of what your pulse rate is (check your neck or wrist areas), take your pulse for 10 seconds, then multiply this number by 6 to get your rate per minute. You can also purchase a pulse-taking monitor for a quick and easy reading.

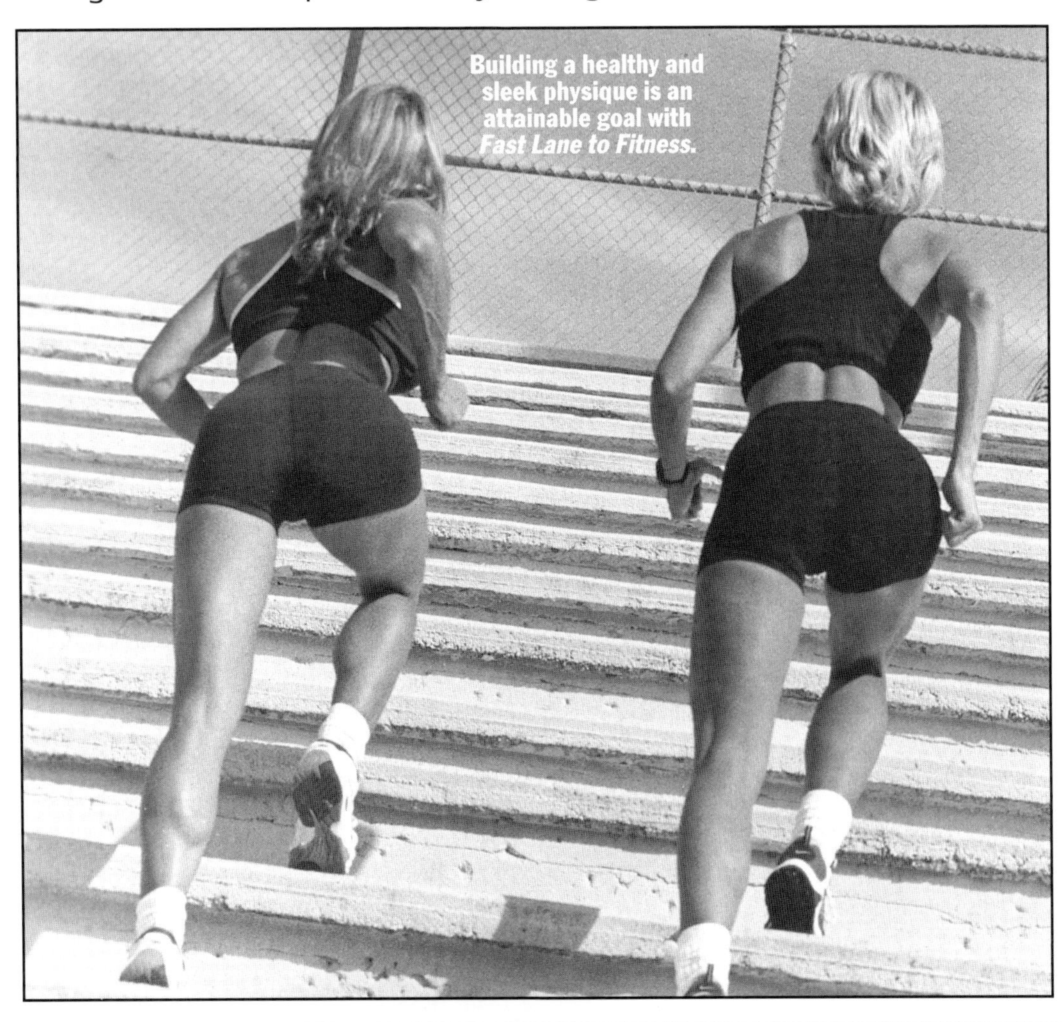

Building a healthy and sleek physique is an attainable goal with *Fast Lane to Fitness.*

To find your exact age and target heart rate you may have to do a small amount of extrapolation if you are not the listed age, but the following table will help you quickly find the heart-rate range you want. Remember, 50 percent is only for beginners; try to move into the 65 to 85 percent range after a few initial workouts. Keep your heartbeat within these ranges by speeding up or slowing down as necessary during the workout. Champion Ironman Mark Allen (*Outside*, February 1997) notes that it is important to stay below your maximum aerobic heart rate throughout your workout. This means not exceeding the listed range for your age.

TARGET HEART-RATE TABLE

Age	50% MHR	65% MHR	75% MHR	85% MHR
20	100	130	150	170
25	98	127	146	166
30	95	124	143	162
35	93	120	139	157
40	90	117	135	153
45	88	114	131	149
50	85	111	128	145
55	83	107	124	140
60	80	104	120	136
65	78	101	116	132
70	75	98	113	128
75	73	94	109	123
80	70	91	105	119

Check your pulse rate fairly often when you are first getting into working out. You will soon learn what pace allows you to stay within your target heart rate for the various aerobic workouts. Learn to make a habit of checking your pulse rate, even after you have been working out for a while. If you don't like the hassle of manually taking your pulse, a digital pulse monitor can be purchased for under $20.

Stay within your target heart range at all times during your aerobic workout.

FAT FUEL RANGE

In addition to your heart rate, there is another important item to be aware of – the level at which your physique starts burning off bodyfat. Your body starts to burn fat for fuel after about 20 minutes of nonstop activity. During the first 20 minutes, the body expends about one-fifth of its glycogen stores. It takes

In order to burn off bodyfat, you have to work out nonstop, for more than 20 minutes in your target heart-rate range. In the first 20 minutes of activity the body primarily uses glycogen for fuel.

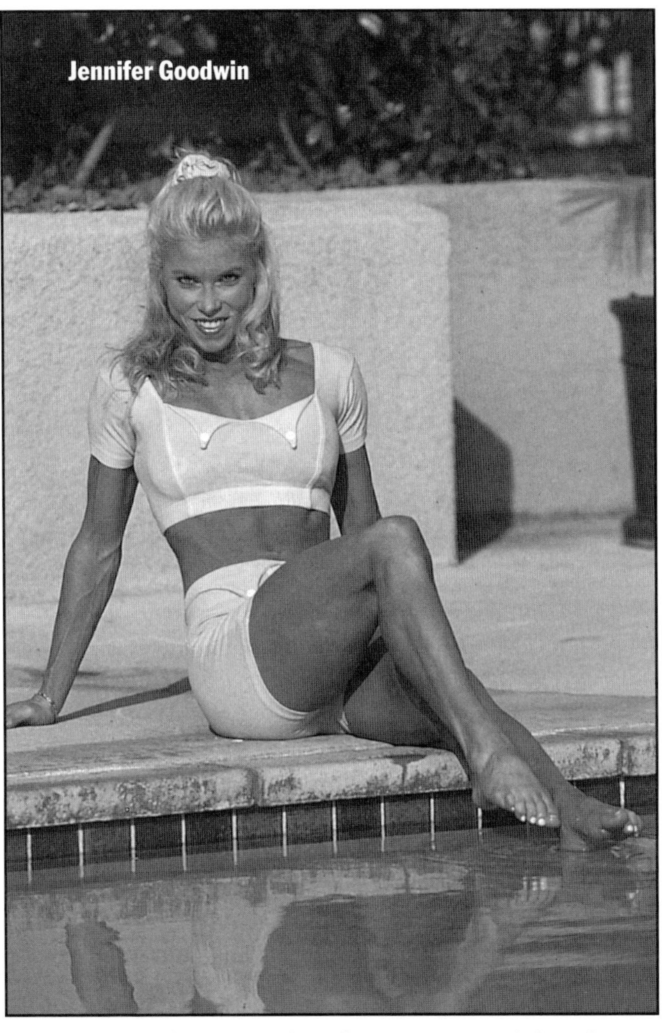
Jennifer Goodwin

time for the fat tissue to be stimulated and release fatty acids to be carried to the muscle cells for use as energy (*Muscle & Fitness*, January 1996). For approximately the first 20 minutes of your workout you are using ATP and glycogen for fuel. This does nothing to get rid of your stored bodyfat. People often run a quick mile, or swim a couple of laps, and think they have accomplished burning off fat. They are wrong! All they have done is blown their ATP and glycogen stores, and have not come near utilizing their bodyfat. Many people don't know this and make the common mistake of not working out long enough with a continuous aerobic exercise. It is important for you to understand this concept if you want to maximize your fitness and health potential. The key to successful aerobic conditioning is to make your workouts last longer than 20 minutes. Memorize this fact. It is an essential part of the *Fast Lane to Fitness* approach to getting in shape.

20-MINUTE RANGE

It is essential you get in a workout that lasts longer than 20 minutes. Note that it is not just 20 minutes, but more than 20 minutes. The 20-minute mark is where you start to burn bodyfat. It is just the beginning point. However, you do not necessarily start at this point. You need to gradually work up to this range. When you begin working out you may be able to go for only 15 minutes, or even less than 10. Don't worry about not being able to go for more than 20 minutes initially. You have to condition your body gradually. You present your physique with a workout it can handle, a workout that provides some challenge, then once you have mastered this challenge a couple of times, you present your body with a workout that is a little more difficult. You gradually work your body up to higher levels instead of trying to do everything at once. It is unsafe to try and accomplish everything at once. You need to let your body become accustomed to the work load. For instance, when you start using an aerobic routine you may be able to only go for 10 to 12 minutes. Stay at this level until you can handle it, then move up to 15 minutes per workout. After 15 minutes, move up to 20. By moving your level of fitness up gradually, you can "step" all the way past 60 minutes, given enough time. The body gradually becomes used to the workout, and you can soon handle smoothly what you could not do earlier. After several workouts, 20 minutes should be no problem. Once you have built your body up to the 20-minute mark, you should seek to go beyond this range. A 30-minute workout means you will have burned off bodyfat for approximately 10 minutes. A 40-minute aerobic workout means you will have burned off bodyfat for approximately 20 minutes. Remember, once you have built a base, working out nonstop for at least 20 minutes, the 20-minute mark becomes your new base minimum. However, for the *Fast Lane to Fitness* approach, the aim is to workout in an aerobic manner for 30 to 45 minutes per workout. If you can get in a workout in this range, you will be burning off bodyfat, increasing your endurance, and your health.

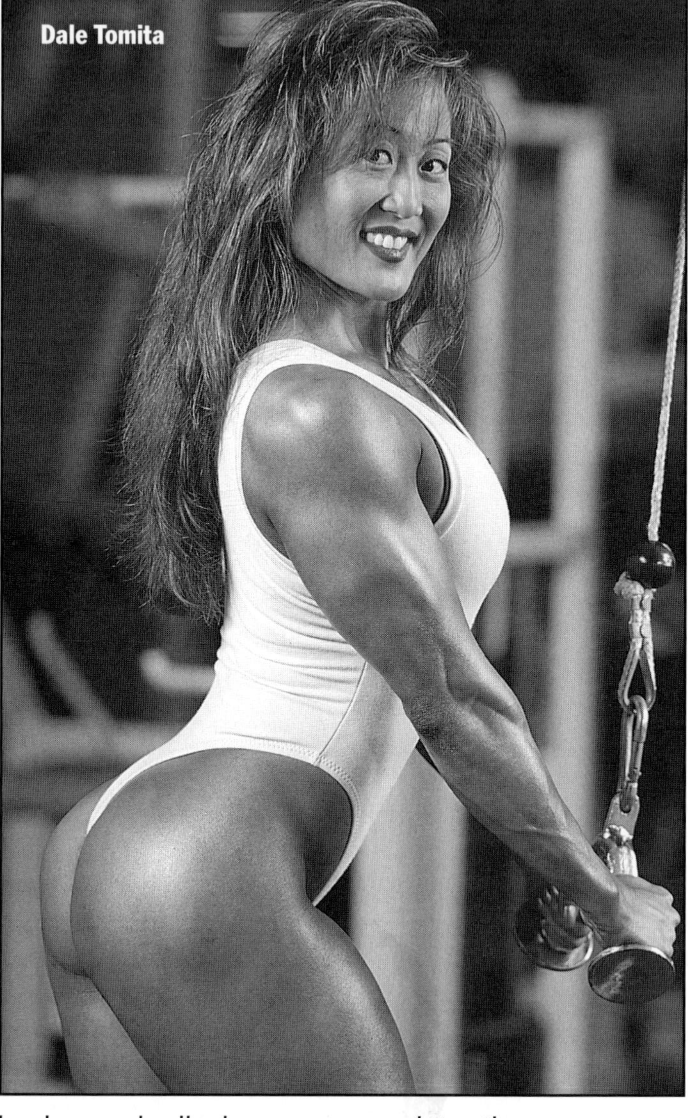
Dale Tomita

The target time range for the *Fast Lane to Fitness* aerobic workout is 30 to 45 minutes.

An occasional longer workout is also a good idea for burning off more fat and increasing your endurance even further. You do not need to go for the really long workouts all of the time – an occasional long workout will do the trick. This program is designed for those who do not have a lot of extra time and therefore the target aerobic workout is set at 30 to 45 minutes. On occasion, when you have the opportunity (and make the opportunity now and then), go for a longer aerobic workout of 45 to 60 minutes. This longer workout will take you to a new level of endurance capabilities, and will also burn off a good deal of bodyfat. It will also make the regular workouts of 30 to 45 minutes seem like a breeze in comparison. For those with tight weekly schedules these longer workouts will be infrequent, but they should still be performed when time permits.

If possible, perform an occasional longer 45- to 60-minute aerobic workout.

NONSTOP MOVEMENT

The aerobic exercise you perform should be nonstop and continuous, from the time you begin the exercise until the time you stop. Instead of using short bursts of energy, you want to make a prolonged effort of endurance. Short bursts of action are not aerobic in nature, don't burn off bodyfat, and don't do much at all for your cardiovascular system. In order to get full aerobic stimulation and benefits, and to burn off bodyfat, your workouts need to be nonstop. Once you start your aerobic workout you need to stick with it until you have completed it. Stop-and-go action won't cut it – the *Fast Lane to Fitness* emphasis is on nonstop movement of the major muscle groups. Don't rest until you are finished with your workout.

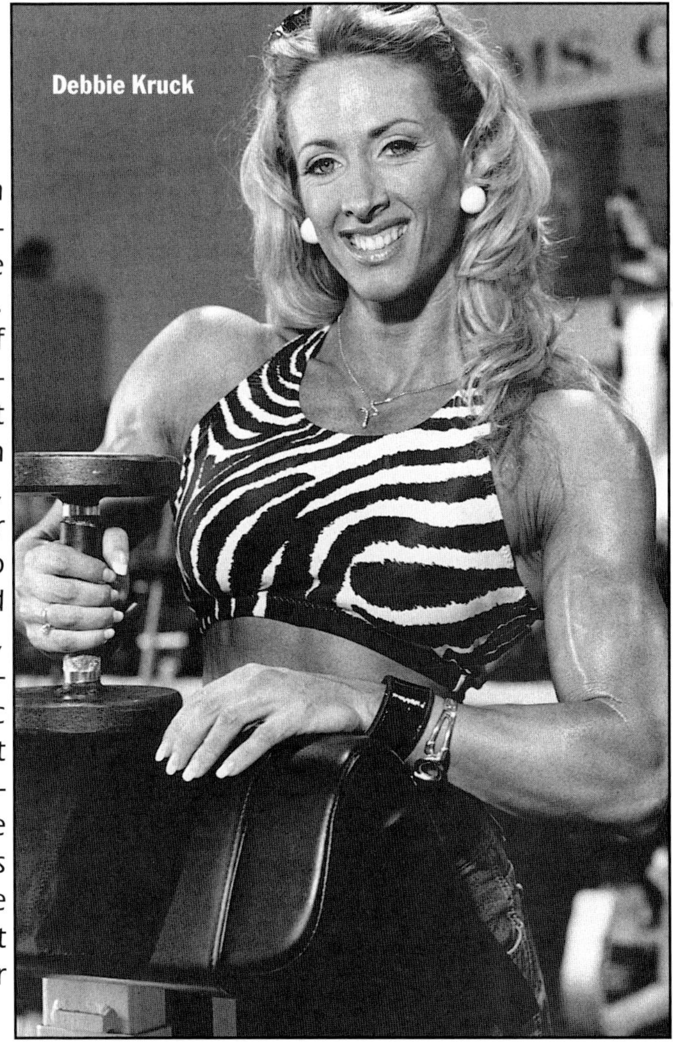
Debbie Kruck

Aerobic training needs to be performed nonstop for the best results.

SLOW START

Start your aerobic workout off slowly. Don't dash off into hard-charging action immediately. Stretch lightly and warmup your body. Mark Allen, the champion Ironman, starts his aerobic workouts by actually walking the first few blocks, and then does a slow mile before he works up to his aerobic threshold (*Outside*, February 1997). If the "most fit man in the world" needs to warm up slowly, so do you. Taking a slow start is a good idea for everyone. It is also a smart idea because your body is using ATP and glycogen during the first few minutes of a workout anyway – the faster you go at first, the more glycogen you burn – and glycogen is not fat! So you are not really benefitting from a fast start. When you work, start slow and easy, working up to a more rapid pace.

It is also a good idea to "cool down" as your workout comes to an end. Don't stop abruptly – ease off, and gradually come to a close. Gradually build into a strong-paced workout, and gradually taper off at the end of your workout. This is the best way to condition your body in the arena of aerobic fitness.

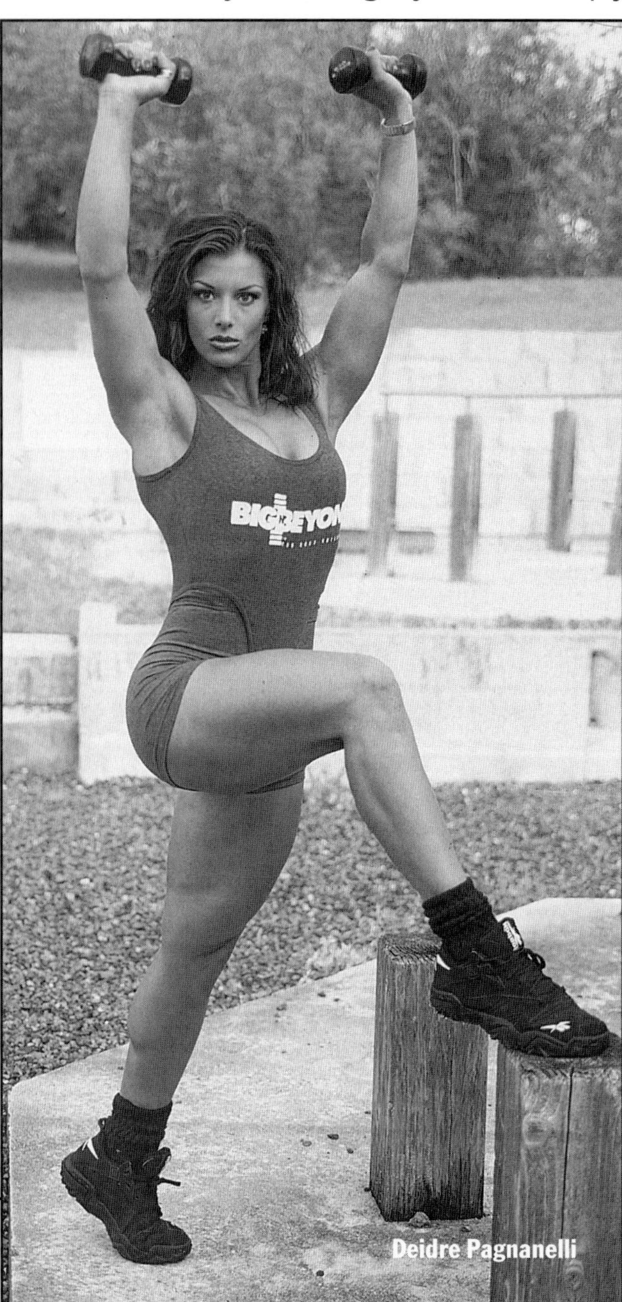

Start your aerobic exercises off slowly, and gradually build up to your target heart-rate range.

MAINTENANCE LEVELS

It is not always possible to get a good 30- to 45-minute aerobic workout in. Time pressures often keep people from this workout. What should you do? skip working out altogether? No way! Some physical activity is better than no

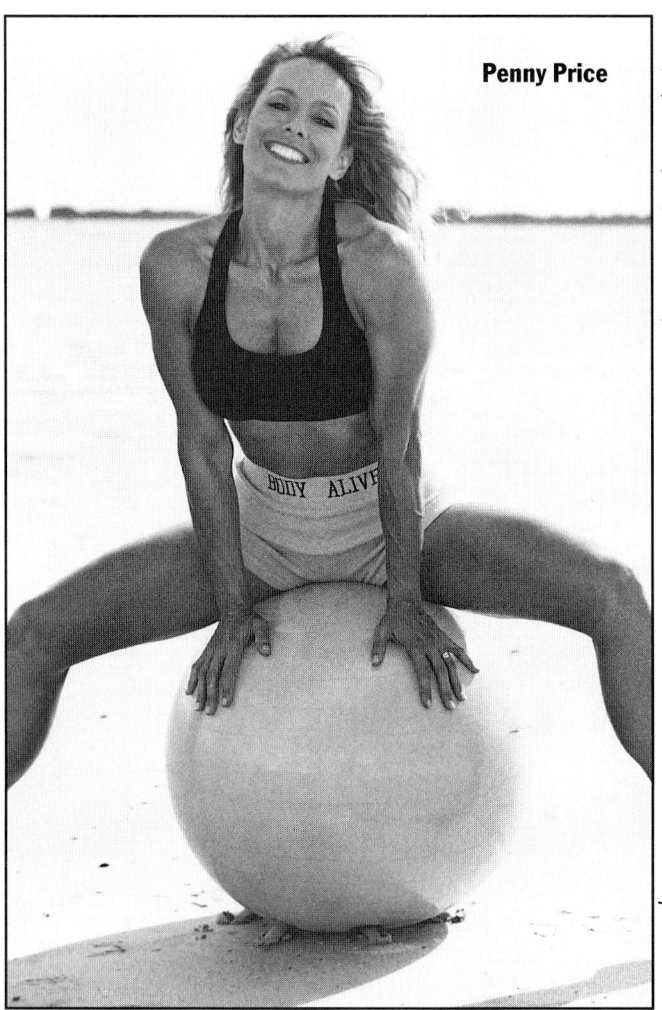

Penny Price

physical activity. Try to get in at least a 20-minute workout. Although you won't burn off a great amount of bodyfat in a 20-minute session, you will maintain your current level of fitness. Ironman athlete Mark Allen notes, "Do I gain anything aerobically (from an occasional 20-minute workout)? No. But I don't want to lose anything either. I've found that if I elevate my heart rate for 10 or 15 minutes, I can maintain what I've already built." (*Outside*, February, 1997). The shorter workout, the one that does not increase your aerobic level or burn fat, at least helps to maintain the level of fitness you are at. It prevents you from losing ground. This is a strong reason why you want to do some exercise, even if it is short, instead of doing nothing. Again, some fitness is always better than no fitness. So don't neglect your fitness just because you do not have a lot of time to work with. Stick with a short workout until you can get in a longer aerobic workout.

A short workout does have some benefit – it helps you maintain your current level of fitness.

FREQUENCY

How often should you perform an aerobic workout? Most fitness experts agree on three to five workouts per week. However, since this program, *Fast Lane to Fitness*, focuses on women who have hectic schedules, a less frequent workout program is much more appropriate as a weekly aerobic goal. Perhaps you cannot get in as many aerobic workouts as someone like Cory Everson, Mia Finnegan or Theresa Hessler; however, you most likely can get in some workouts. For those on a busy schedule, getting in two to three workouts a week is a good goal to aim for. You can attain a fairly good level of aerobic fitness on two or three workouts per week. These workouts should fall within the 30- to 45-minute-per-workout range. Even one workout a week is better than nothing, even if it is only a 20-minute maintenance workout. Perhaps you can only squeeze in a 20-minute aerobic workout during the week. If this occurs, try to get in a 40- to 45-minute workout on the weekend. Keep your fitness "drive" alive by getting in at least one workout a week. If you miss a week or so, don't quit altogether – simply get back to the program as soon as possible. The body bounces back quite well, and you can catch up to where you were in no time at all.

Try to get in two or three aerobic workouts a week. If you are unable to, keep your fitness "drive" alive by getting in at least one workout a week.

It should be possible for most people to find some extra time here and there to get in a couple of workouts. If you organize and plan your week right you may be able to find some time for a few workouts. Planning ahead and keeping some workout gear with you in the office, or car, keeps you prepared for the opportunity to attain an increased level of fitness.

EXERCISE CHOICES

When it comes to aerobic exercise you have a wide variety of choices. There are dozens and dozens of possibilities, and people seem to keep coming up with more. Since you are in a hurry, there is no need to learn some new and exotic fitness movement. The basic favorites work very well for the purpose of aerobic fitness and burning off bodyfat. The basic movements of the larger muscle groups (walking, running, hiking, climbing, etc.) can be used to get in an excellent aerobic workout. *Fast Lane to Fitness* utilizes the basic exercises that are known to produce results. The exercises touted in *Fast Lane to Fitness* for aerobic conditioning are also relatively inexpensive to do; some cost nothing at all. There is no need to spend a lot of money to get into great shape.

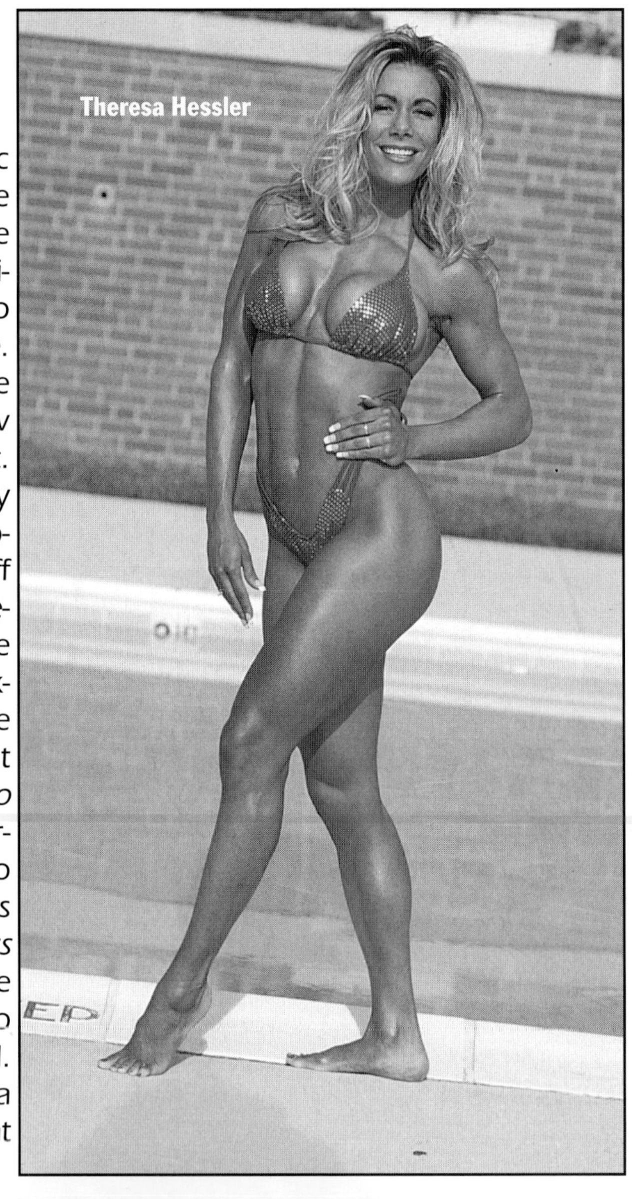
Theresa Hessler

JOGGING

Jogging is a good way to get in an aerobic workout, particularly if you start off slow, and work up to the level where your heart rate is in the target training zone for your age. The one caveat with jogging is to not use it as your sole aerobic workout. Running all of the time, particularly on hard surfaces, can cause injury to your legs and feet. If you do choose to use jogging as an aerobic workout, mix it in with other exercises.

POWER WALKING

Power walking is a great way to increase your level of fitness. Power walking can be performed by almost everyone. Power walking involves very brisk walking – at a pace that is about as fast a walk as you can take. Power walking is not strolling – it is moving along at a good clip, anywhere from 3 to 5 miles per hour. You can find your speed by noting how long it takes you to cover a mile. A local track proves useful for finding your average power-walking speed. Most tracks are a quarter-mile in length. Time yourself as you make four laps. If you can cover four laps in 15 minutes, you are moving at a speed of 4 miles per hour. If you can cover four laps in 12 minutes, you are going 5 miles per hour. If you take 20 minutes to get in four laps, you are going 3 miles per hour. A good pace for most people to maintain is 4 miles per hour; not everyone can do this, so the minimum is 3 miles per hour. If you can get in the 5-mile-per-hour range you are really moving along.

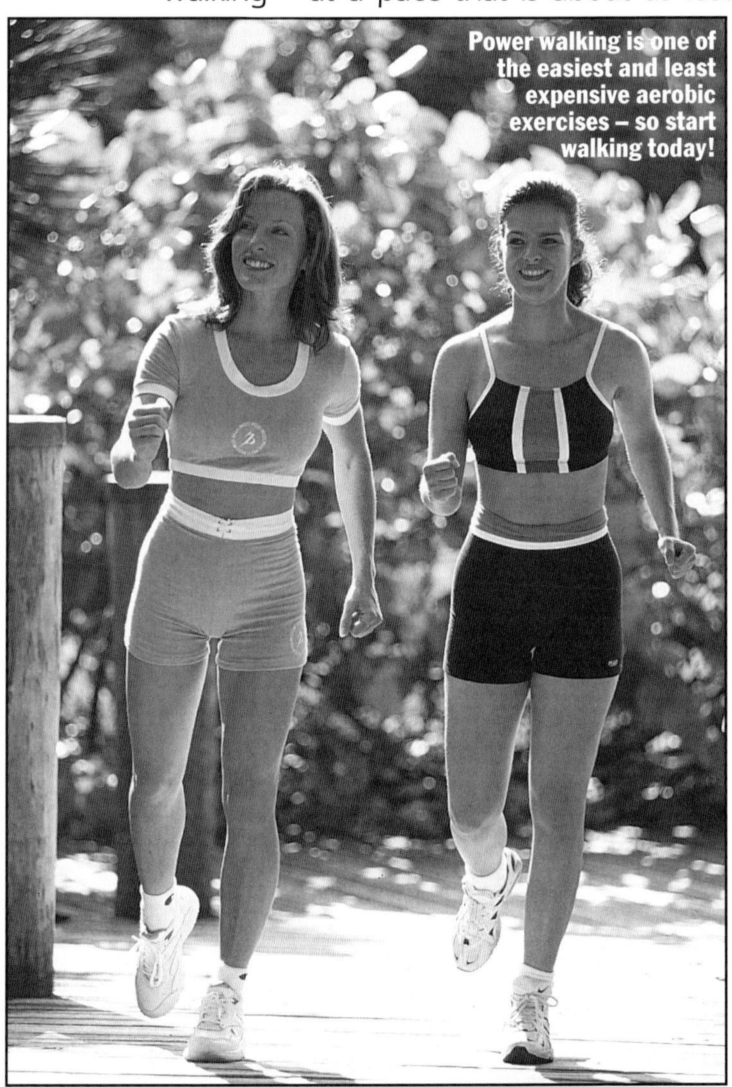

Power walking is one of the easiest and least expensive aerobic exercises – so start walking today!

Continual running and jumping on hard surfaces can cause injury.

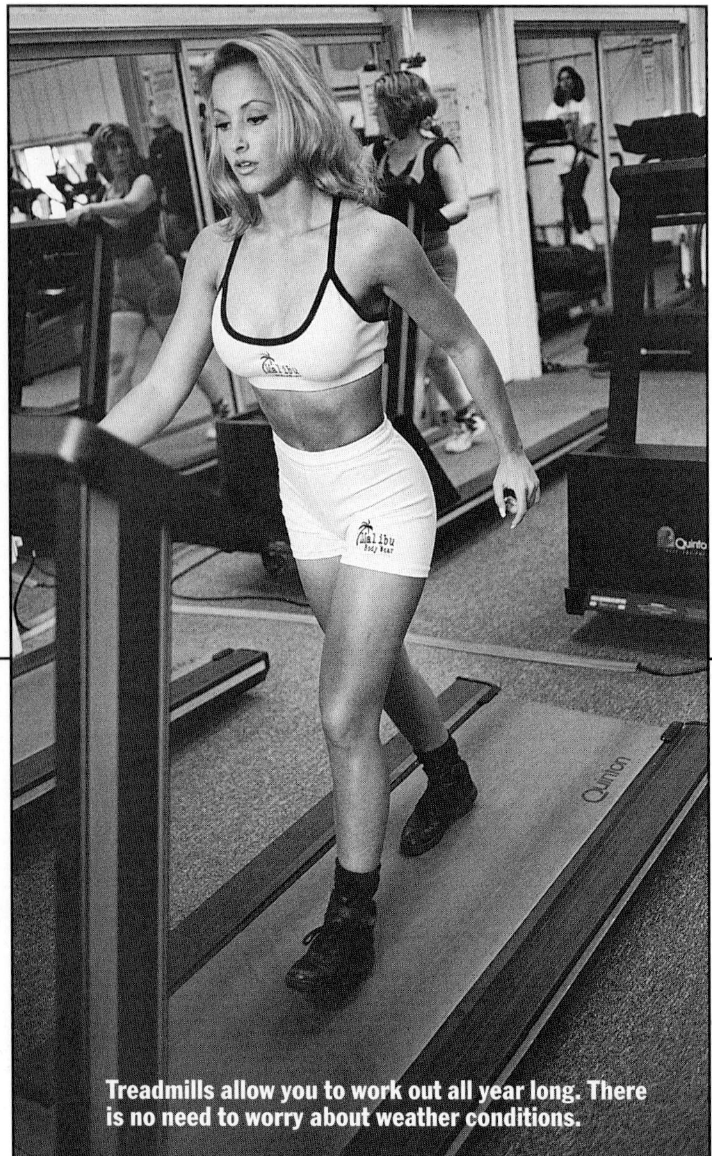

Treadmills allow you to work out all year long. There is no need to worry about weather conditions.

More people are starting to become interested in this excellent conditioning exercise. One study noted that "people over 65 who walk more than four hours per week are 30 percent less likely to be hospitalized for heart disease than sedentary people of the same age. Walking can also have positive effects on blood pressure, bodyweight, and cholesterol levels" (*Quest,* winter 1997).

TREADMILL

The treadmill is a variation of power walking. The treadmill allows you to move a bit quicker, and many have added incline capabilities. This allows you to burn more calories during your workout because the incline makes you work harder. The steeper the incline, the more fat you burn. However, it is a good idea to start at a lower level, moving up to a more challenging workout. The treadmill is a popular machine and most gyms have several available. You can also purchase one fairly inexpensively at a local sporting-goods store. You can enhance your time on the treadmill by listening to a cassette tape or by watching television. If you do so, your workout will go by quickly. Using a treadmill for your aerobic exercise is fantastic for continual fitness because it allows you to work out all year long since you do not have to worry about weather (or dogs). Consider this item from the health newsletter *Quest*:

Among indoor workout equipment, the treadmill provides the most efficient way to burn calories – it's up to 40 percent more effective than other machines (*The Journal of the American Medical Association)*. Treadmills induce higher rates of energy expenditure and aerobic demands than a stationary cycle, rowing machine, stair stepper or cross-country skiing simulator.

STAIR CLIMBING

Stair climbing, or stair stepping, is a great conditioning tool. The stair-stepping machine has become quite popular at fitness clubs, and home versions sell well too. Stair stepping can also be done on regular stairs if you have access to them, and this type of stair stepping costs nothing. Or you can use a simple one-step platform, stepping up and down repeatedly. Stair climbing works the leg muscles to a substantial degree, in addition to promoting aerobic conditioning and burning off bodyfat. Stair stepping is a premium aerobic exercise.

Stair climbing is a fantastic way to burn off bodyfat.

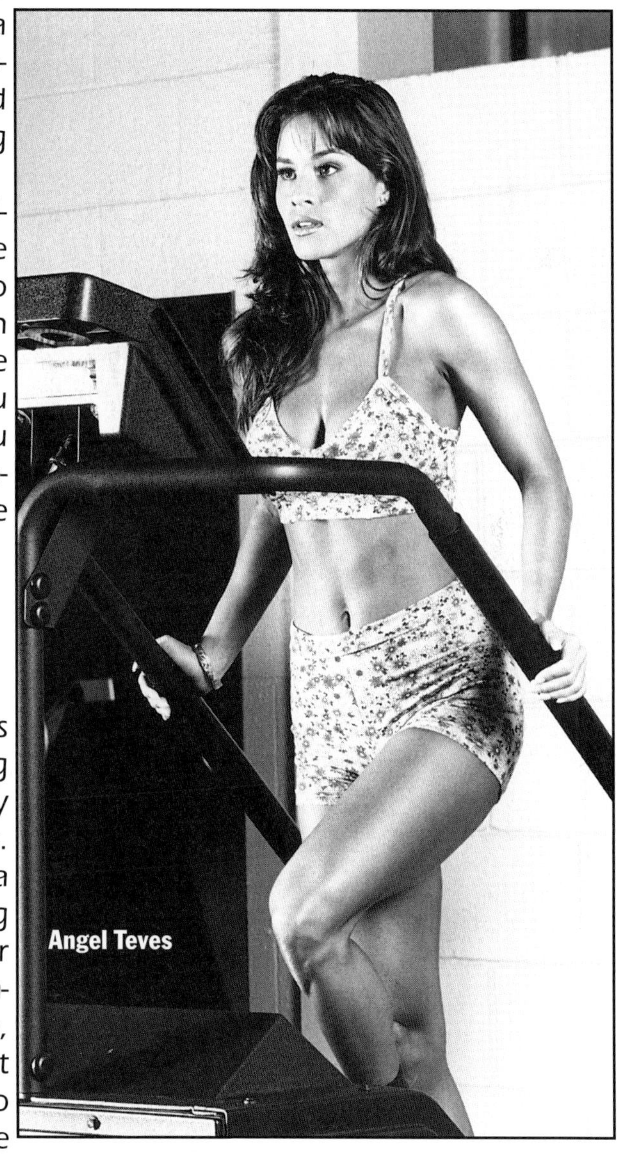

Angel Teves

Mini-stair steppers are available at a very reasonable price (around $20). They are also portable, so you can take them on trips if you travel frequently. These small stair-stepping units allow you to get in a good workout while you are on the move or at home, especially if you only have a small space to work out in.

BIKING

Biking is another exercise that works well for aerobic conditioning. Biking can be performed with a stationary bike or with a regular bike outdoors. Both types allow you to spend a prolonged amount of time using your leg muscles to condition your body. Biking, whether with the stationary bike or an outdoor bike, should be performed in a constant pedaling manner – not stop-and-go or "coasting." Check your heart rate to make sure you are working hard enough to keep your heart beat in the target training zone (see the table on page 24). Biking outside can provide for a peaceful workout, especially if you live close to a park or decide to ride some bike trails.

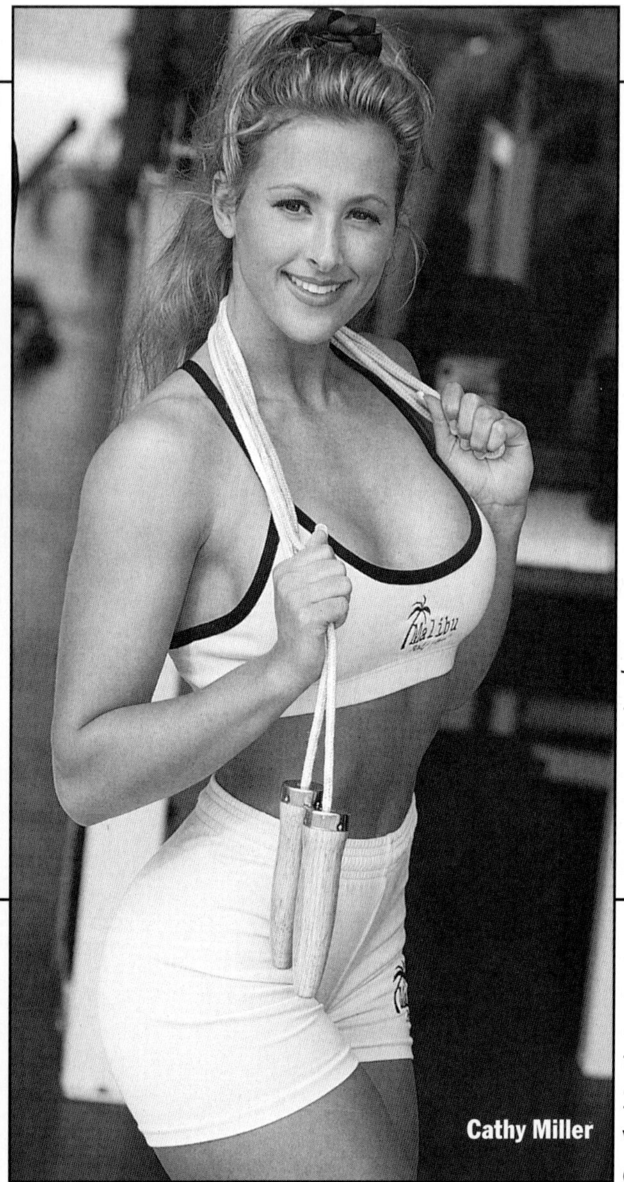

Cathy Miller

JUMPING ROPE

Jumping rope is a great way to get in a strong aerobic workout. It is important, however, not to jump on a surface that is too hard (such as concrete) as this can cause shin splints. Jump rope on a surface that is firm but has some give. You can make a jumping platform with a few boards and a small piece of carpet. Jumping rope is an intense aerobic workout, and helps build body coordination and leg strength. Jumping rope is super inexpensive, and can be done at home or on the road (by taking a jump rope and sweats with you when you travel). Jumping rope is a great way to add variety to your training program.

NORDIC SKIING

Nordic skiing, both the outdoor and indoor types (such as the popular Nordic Track) have long been known to be great for aerobic conditioning. Some people favor this type of aerobic workout, and like to get into the cross-country groove. Nordic skiing provides for spectacular scenery when performed outside – but watch out for an avalanche! If you are in an area where there is significant snow in the winter, instead of getting "cabin fever," get out and burn off some of those holiday calories with some cross-country skiing. Or you may have a cross-country skiing simulator and can perform your workout indoors.

CHOOSE YOUR FAVORITE

The exercises that have been featured are just a few of the more popular aerobic choices available. You can use one of these or perhaps you favor an exercise that hasn't been mentioned. There are many new fitness machines entering the market on a continual basis (such as the HealthRider, etc.) and most of them work well. The key factor with any exercise is to make sure it brings your heart rate into the target training range, and keeping it there throughout the entire workout. This is easily accomplished when the exercise works one or more of the major muscle groups for a nonstop workout of sufficient length. To realize the full potential of the workout make it last for more than 20 minutes.

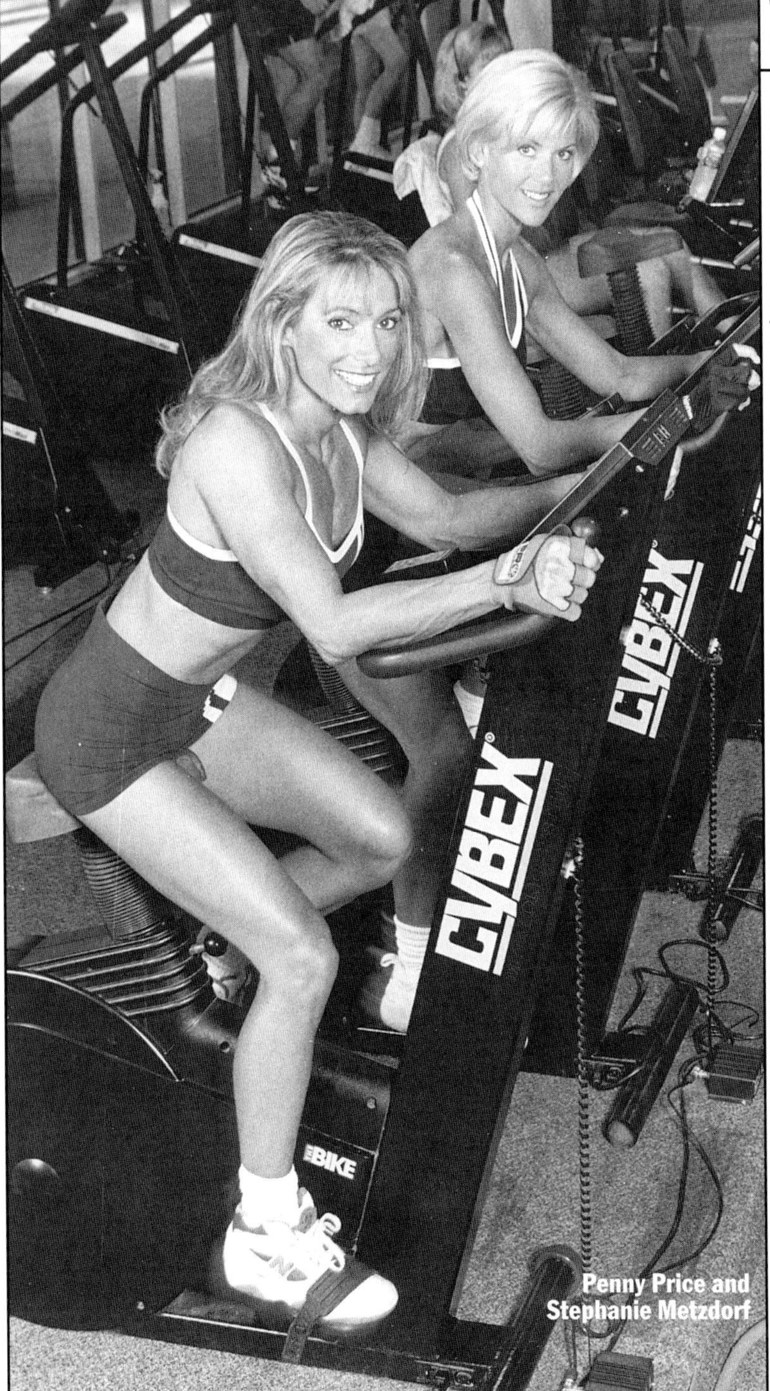

Penny Price and Stephanie Metzdorf

VARIETY

Rotating different aerobic exercises can make each workout interesting and continually challenging.

There is nothing that says you are stuck with only one type of aerobic workout. Try different aerobic exercises. You may discover you like something new and challenging. It will also help you become well-rounded in the fitness sphere. Physique star Nikki Fuller states that in training for a contest she uses a variety of different aerobic exercises, sometimes several different types in one workout! (*Flex*, January 1993). Rotating different exercises keeps you motivated and challenges your body in different ways.

A good idea for variation is to use the same workouts during the week and a different aerobic exercise on the weekends. Or yet another idea is to use one type of aerobic exercise for a few weeks or months, then switch to another type for the next few weeks or months. In this manner you can check out a variety of aerobic exercises and discover which ones work well for you, and which don't. Try not to become stuck with only one aerobic exercise unless you really enjoy it. Experiment to find out which exercises have the greatest impact on your body.

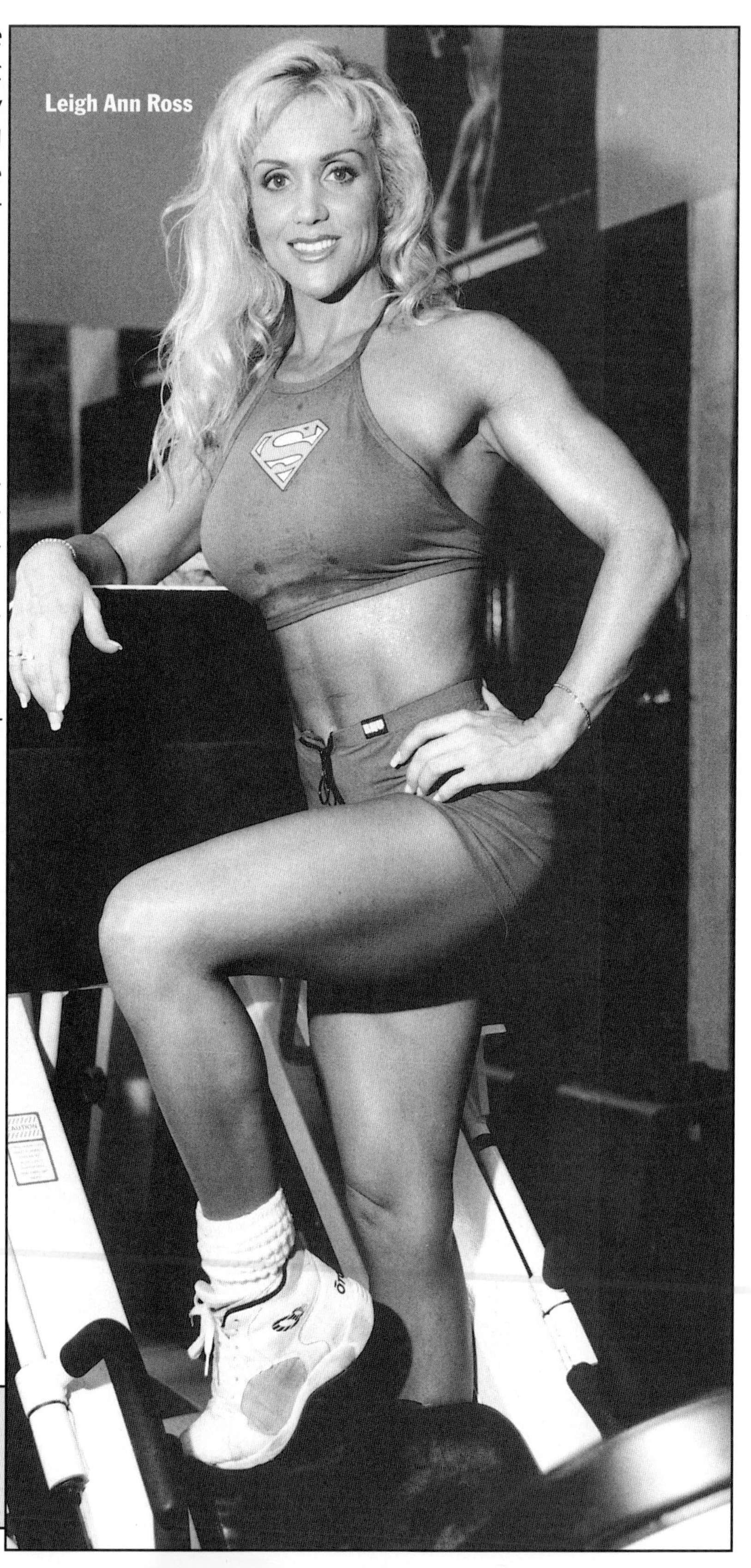
Leigh Ann Ross

ESSENTIAL ELEMENT

The aerobic element of fitness is probably the most essential element of any fitness program. It is crucial to the well-being of your body. You cannot afford to neglect the aerobic conditioning aspect of the *Fast Lane to Fitness* program. Additionally, aerobic conditioning builds endurance and burns off bodyfat, trimming your physique to a lean and mean condition. Aerobic conditioning is a fantastic medium for changing your body. Even if you can only get in a minimal amount of aerobic conditioning, do what you can. Some fitness is better than no fitness, and some aerobic conditioning is far better than none. Make room in your schedule for this important type of exercise.

References

1. "Cardio (Aerobics)," *Muscle & Fitness* (November 1996), 103.
2. "Cardio (Aerobics)," 103.

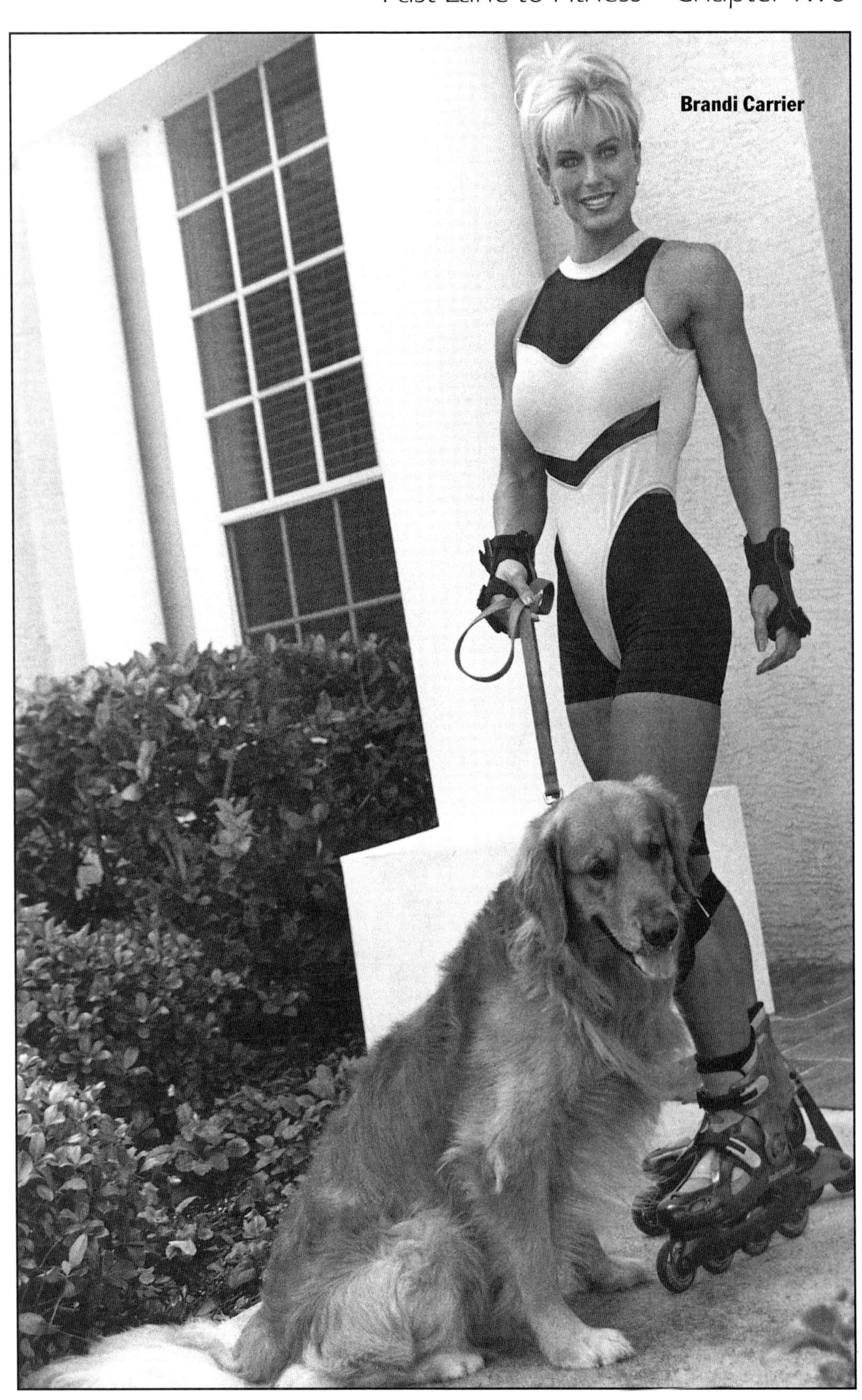

Brandi Carrier

Strength and Shape Training

Aerobic training is one of the essential elements of total fitness. One of the other essential elements is strength and shape training. Aerobic training has a different effect on the body than does strength and shape training; however, both contribute to a healthier and more shaplier physique. Neither should be neglected for optimal conditioning.

Many people are starting to recognize the benefits of adding strength and shape training to their workout mix. One fitness company, SOLOFLEX, points out the benefits of strength and shape training in their *Magic of Strength Training* booklet:

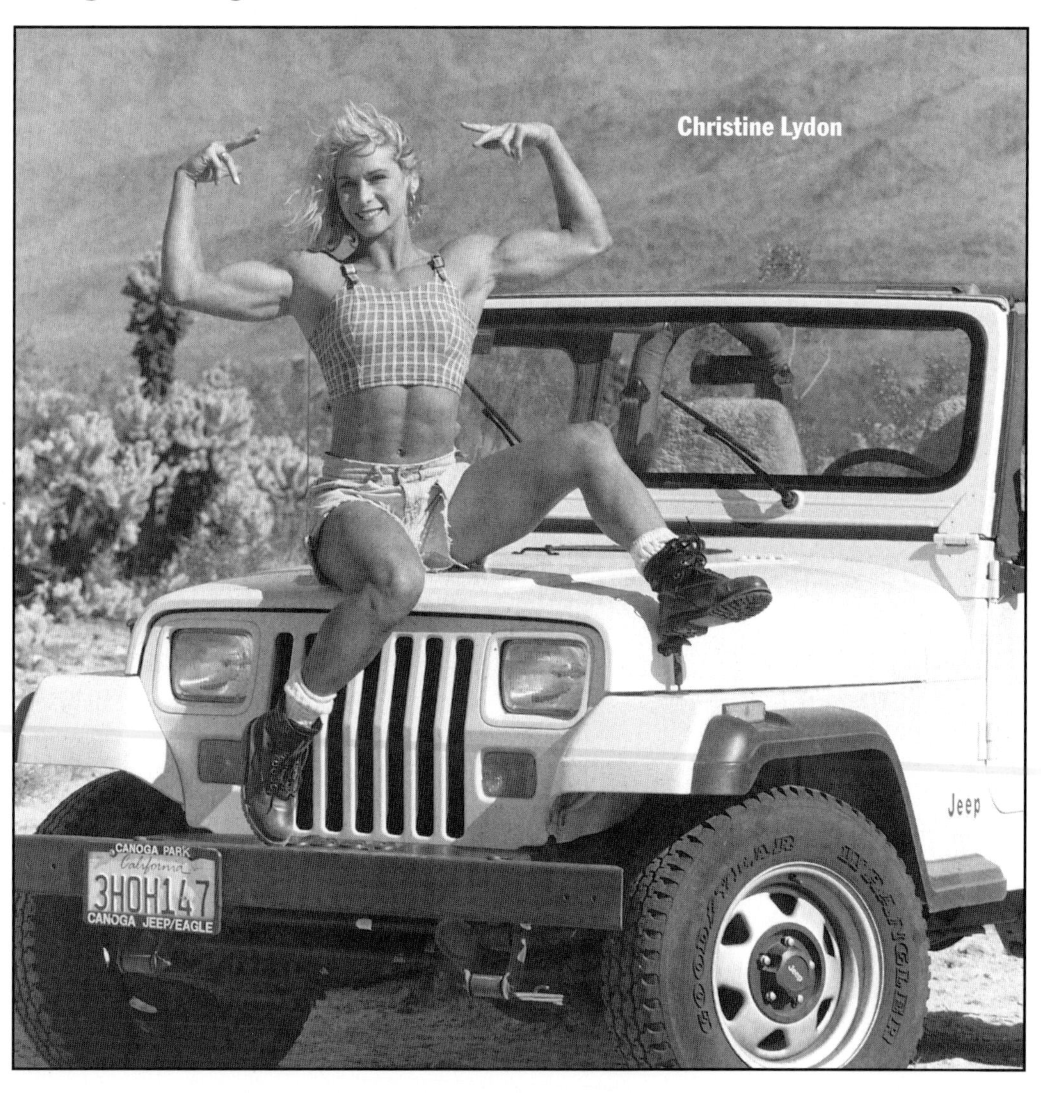

Christine Lydon

No other exercise can do what strength training does for you. It:

1. Increases your metabolism to burn fat.
2. Makes you physically younger.
3. Builds stronger bones.
4. Gives you a better shape.
5. Strengthens your immune system.
6. Makes you more resistant to injury.
7. Lowers blood sugar and cholesterol.
8. Gives you more energy.
9. Makes you feel better, more positive.

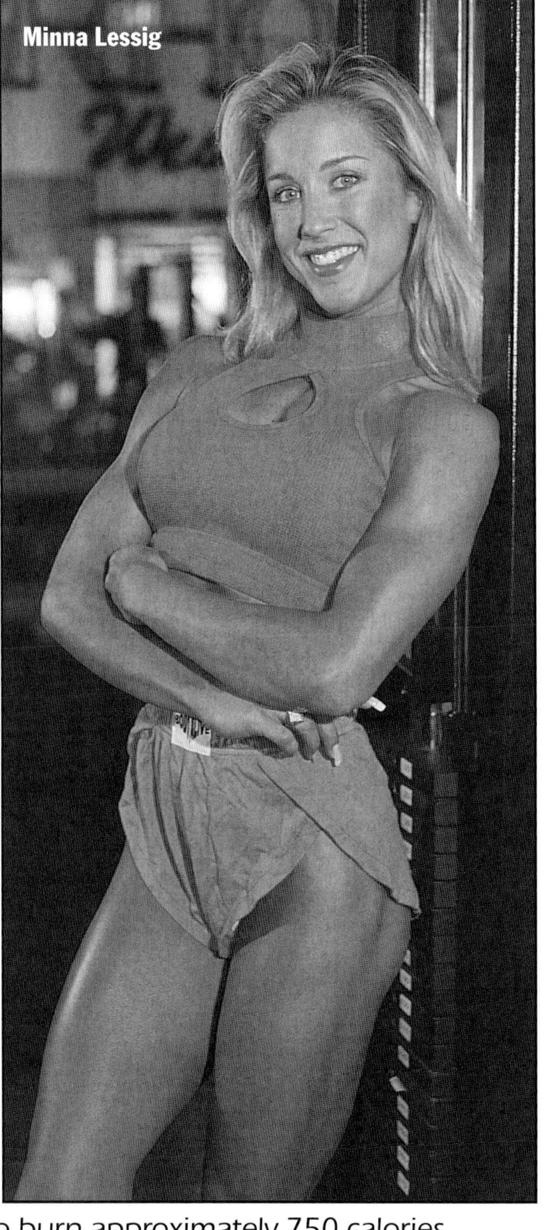
Minna Lessig

As you can see, there are many fantastic reasons for strength and shape training. It is the quickest way to change your appearance in a positive manner. One of the best benefits is that it increases your metabolism to burn fat. This metabolic elevation works throughout the day, not just when you are working out. The SOLOFLEX booklet also points out that "Muscle is three times more dense than fat. To lose fat and slim down permanently you've got to build muscle. The muscle you build will increase your metabolism. In just a short time you can easily build enough muscle to burn an extra 500 to 750 calories every day, at rest. You'd have to spend 2 hours or more on a treadmill to burn 750 calories!"

Strength and shape training is an awesome tool if you're looking to positively change your physique, especially for the busy person. As noted in the SOLOFLEX booklet, you would have to spend 2 hours – or more – on a treadmill to burn approximately 750 calories whereas you could increase your metabolism through the additional muscle you add from strength and shape training to a point where it would automatically burn the extra 750 calories. That's not bad, considering most people don't even spend close to 2 hours or more per day on aerobic training. Most people don't spend that much time on aerobic workouts in one week. Strength and shape training stacks up very well to aerobic training in regards to burning bodyfat. SOLOFLEX is

Strength and shape training is the quickest way to positively change your appearance.

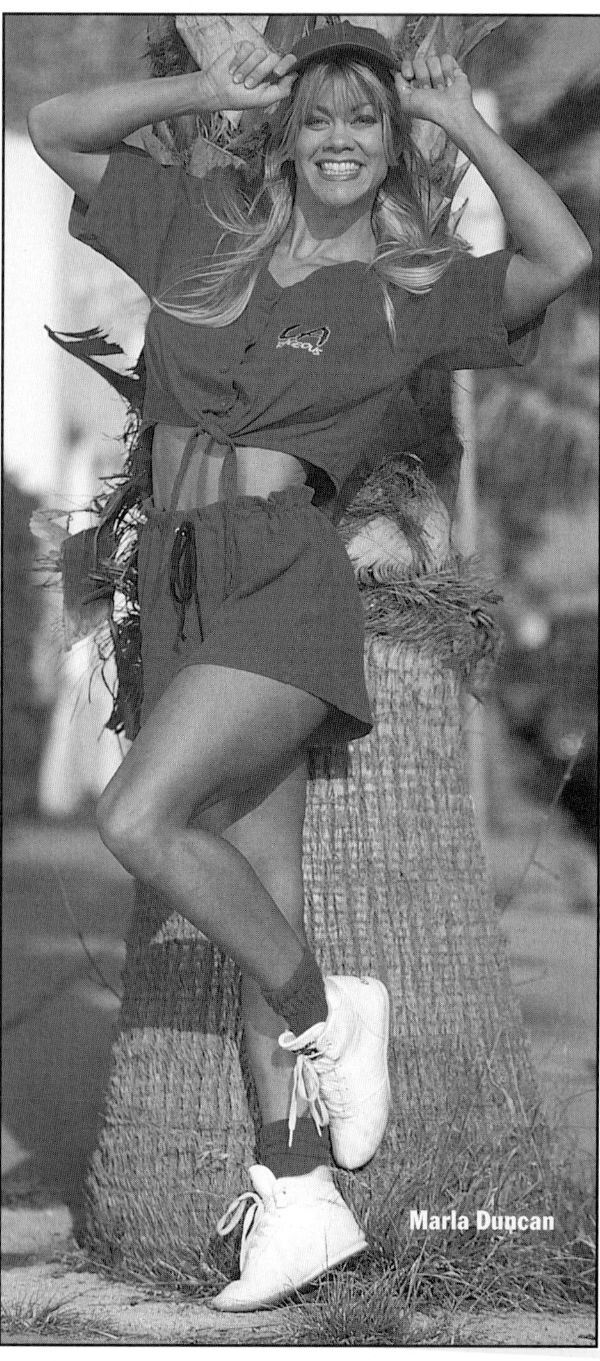
Marla Duncan

not the only one to point out the incredible fat-burning properties of strength and shape training. An article by Todd Balf in *Outside* (February 1997) notes, "Depending on its duration and intensity, a good endurance workout will elevate your metabolism for anywhere from one to six hours. After an hour-long weight-training session, by contrast, your metabolic rate will remain higher for a full 24 hours, thanks to the huge caloric demands of rebuilding muscle tissue. Hoisting the iron is essential to helping you avoid that spare tire."

Strength and shape training rapidly changes the body because the muscles are being built up. In this process the metabolism is fired up to a high degree. Significant change occurs to the physique, change that cannot happen in any other manner. Strength and shape training brings certain unique characteristics to the total fitness mix. Top fitness stars such as Marla Duncan, Laurie Donnelly, Penny Price and hundreds of others use strength and shape training to assist them in getting "the look" – a physique that is trim, sleek and shapely.

THE IMPORTANCE OF STRENGTH AND SHAPE TRAINING

Aerobic conditioning is essential for fitness, but by itself it is incomplete for total fitness. When you use aerobic exercise you are primarily conditioning your heart and respiratory systems and burning off bodyfat (and building your body's endurance levels). This is great for trimming (subtracting body size), but it does not do a lot for shaping. Total conditioning should involve both trimming and shaping. And aerobic conditioning is also incomplete in that it only produces endurance, not pure power strength. Aerobic fitness does increase strength levels, but only by a minimal amount. To significantly affect strength and to cause a reshaping of the body, more is needed. That is where specific strength and shape training comes in. In order to produce strength and shape changes you need to use definite strength and shape exercises, which are vastly different from endurance work.

Aerobic conditioning is important, but it is only part of the fitness mix. By itself, it is incomplete. Strength and shaping exercises are also essential elements for total fitness.

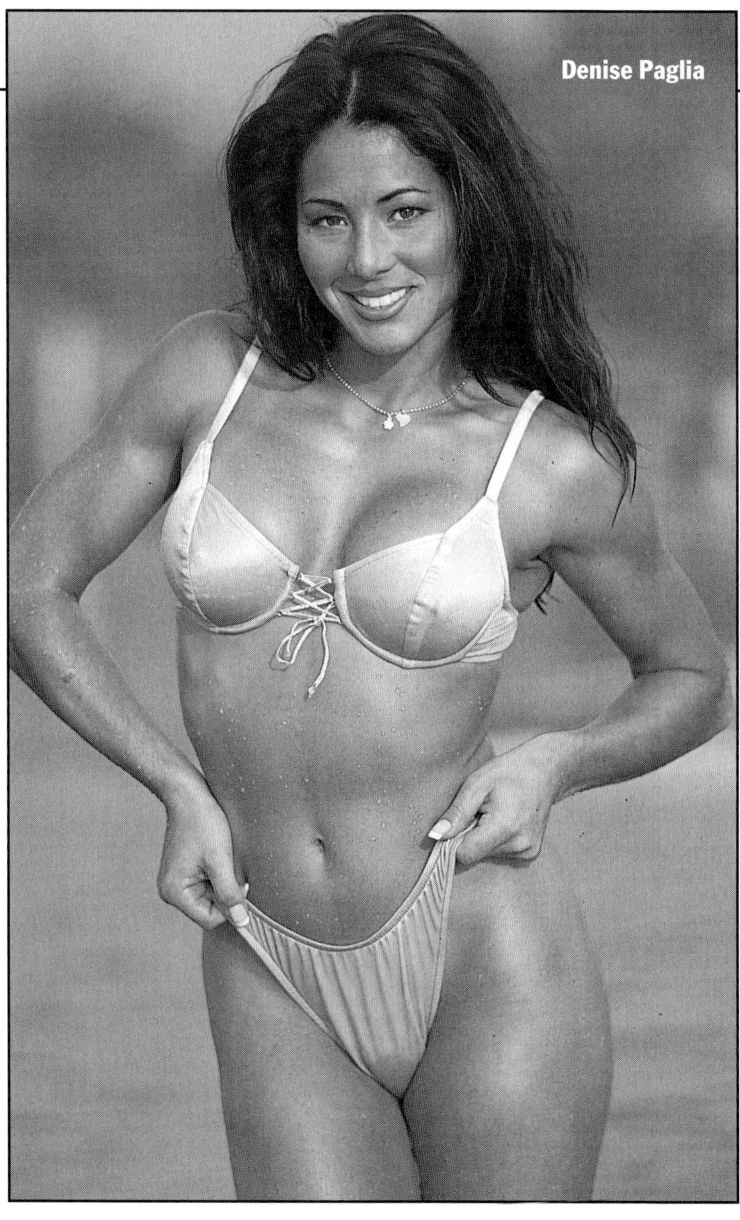
Denise Paglia

BASIC DIFFERENCES

As mentioned in the last chapter, aerobic exercises are aerobic (with air), where oxygen is involved in the metabolic process that produces the energy involved. Additionally, aerobic exercise uses both glycogen and fat for fuel, first using glycogen, then switching to fat. The process of aerobic action occurs with sustained effort for a long period of time at a low level of intensity (as contrasted with the high level of intensity of anaerobic effort). On the other hand, anaerobic means "without air," and consists of short bursts of intense effort, fueled primarily by ATP stored in the muscles (this source lasts only a few seconds) and glycogen. Anaerobic activity is short in nature because your body cannot sustain the high level of energy and activity over a long period of time, and your fuel source (ATP and glycogen) tapers off after a while.

The nature of aerobic exercise is such that it works best for increasing endurance, and burning off bodyfat in the immediate workout. The nature of strength and shape training is such that it works best for adding strength and power, and burning off bodyfat, not in the immediate workout, but afterwards. Each type of workout conditions the body in a unique manner. Each is necessary for total body training.

DENSE AND INTENSE WORKOUTS

Can a strength and shaping routine be added to a busy person's schedule? Yes. It is possible to get in a good strength and shaping workout in a short period of time. The adage of the earlier chapter remains true – some fitness is better than no fitness. Some strength and shaping exercise is far better than none at all.

The very nature of strength and shaping exercises lends itself well to a brief workout. The best strength and shaping environment is an intense and brief environment. For the busy person a quick and focused workout is required, and in fact most exercises should be brief and focused. That is how you best stimulate the body for gains. A "dense and intense" workout, pack-

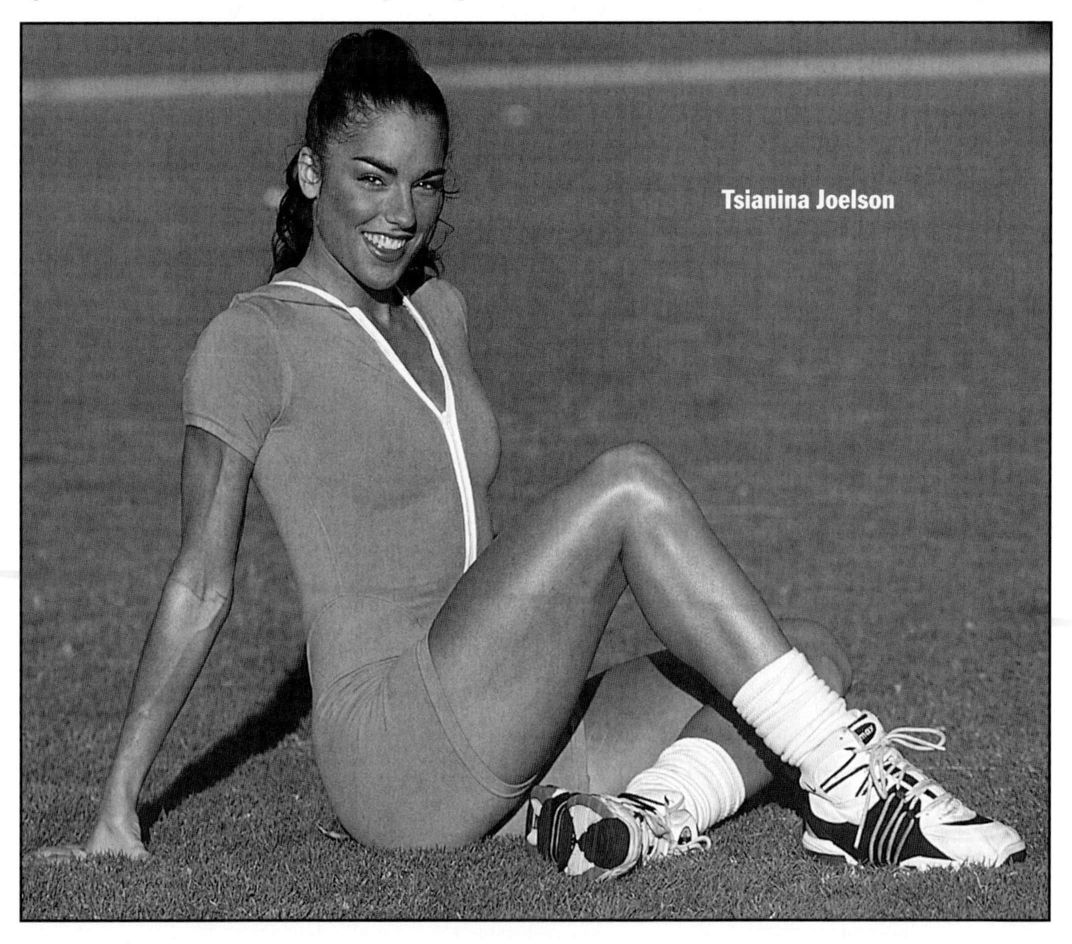

Tsianina Joelson

ing a good deal of training into a short amount of time, works wonders for achieving the aims of a stronger and well-shaped body.

TWO TYPES

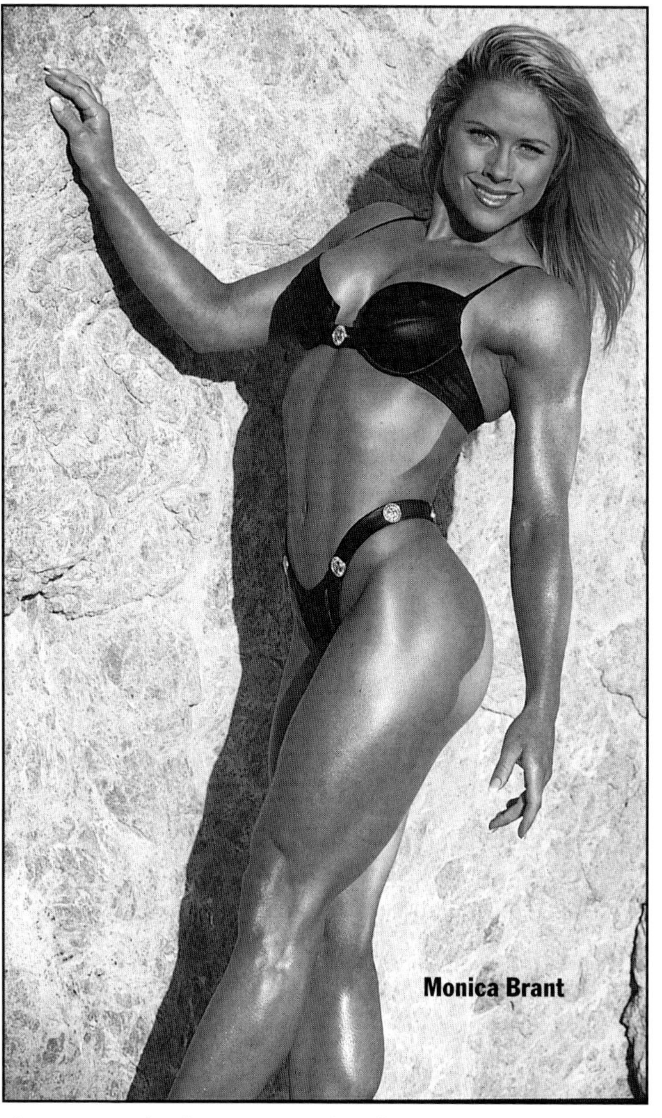
Monica Brant

There are two basic types of strength and shaping exercises, freehand exercise and weight training. Freehand exercises primarily rely upon using your bodyweight to condition your body, while weight training uses various types of weights. Both work well but weight training is the superior of the two. With freehand exercises you can only progress to a certain level – the amount of repetitions per exercise you can perform at bodyweight. With weight training you can use a variety of different weight levels. Freehand exercises are also pretty much restricted to the large muscle groups, working them in a compound manner (using a couple of the major muscle groups together). With weight training you can get more specific with your training and work smaller bodyparts as well as the larger muscle groups. Weights allow you various options besides changing the weight level; you can use the weight in the form of a barbell, dumbell, or machine. Weight training allows you to concentrate on one area at a time (for example the right arm) through the use of dumbells. All things considered, weight training is the most effective manner in which to provide the physique with strength- and shape-training results. It is the most productive manner in which to significantly change the body.

For *Fast Lane to Fitness*, both types of strength and shaping exercises will be featured. You may not have access to a gym or home weight equipment, therefore freehand exercises may be the best route for you. On the other hand, if you do have access to weights (barbells, dumbells, or machines), by all means take advantage of them.

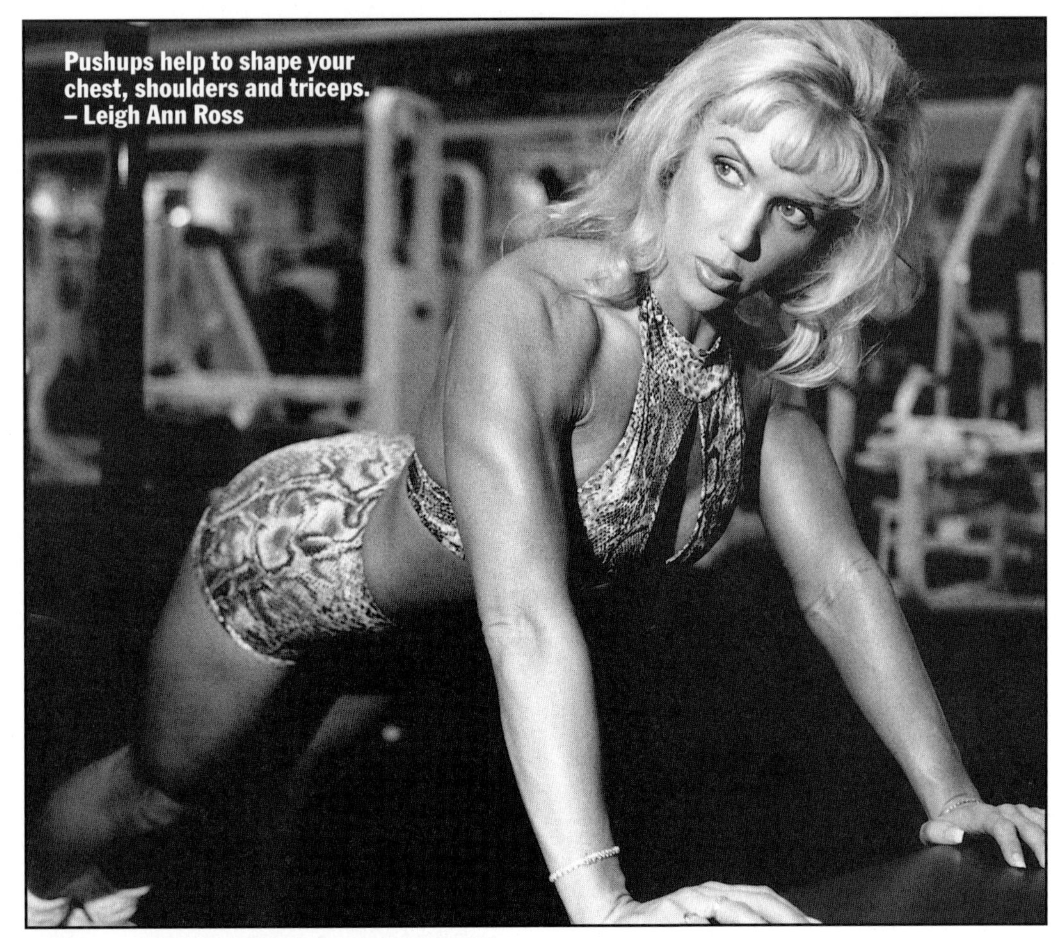
Pushups help to shape your chest, shoulders and triceps. – Leigh Ann Ross

FAST FREEHAND EXERCISES

A few of the top freehand exercises can be used to really add strength and shape to your physique.

PUSHUPS

The pushup is performed by assuming a face-down position on the floor, arms and feet holding the body up (note – if regular pushups are too difficult, use your knees instead of your feet for rear stabilization). Your hands should be about shoulder width apart or a little wider. Lower yourself until you lightly touch the floor, then push yourself back to a full extension. This exercise will strengthen and shape your chest, triceps and frontal shoulder region.

DIPS

The dip exercise is performed by positioning your body between two level and stable surfaces, or on a dip bar. Extend your arms so that they support your body, making sure not to lock out completely, then lower your body slowly. Your body should be rigid except for your arms, which should be doing all of the work. Dips work your triceps, shoulders, and chest muscles.

CHINS

The medium-grip chinup is the final upper-body movement. Grasp a chinup bar with an underhand grip (palms facing you) with your hands approximately shoulder width apart. Perform a full chinup, bringing your chin over the bar, then lowering yourself. Not everyone can perform chinups, particularly in the initial stages of training. Sometimes the use of a chair can help. Physique star Nikki Fuller uses a chair or something else to put her feet on as a "spotting mechanism" (*MuscleMag International*, June 1994). A good substitute for the regular chinup is the Gravitron machine, which assists in performing the full movement. If you can perform chinups without help, great; if not, use a chair to help, or use the Gravitron machine. Medium-grip chinups work your biceps and back.

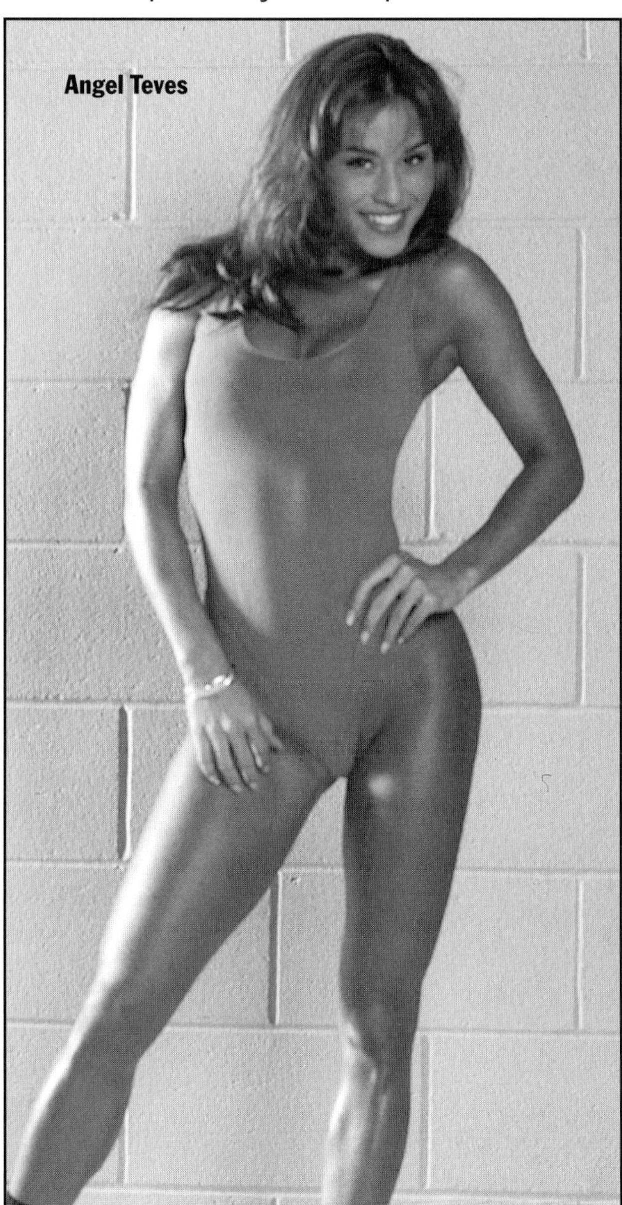
Angel Teves

That's all of the exercises for the upper body – just three. Remember, this is the *Fast Lane to Fitness*.

SINGLE-LEG SQUATS

For the lower body, a couple of freehand exercises are used. One is the single-leg squat. The single-leg squat is performed by steadying your body with one or two hands and squatting down on one leg. Keep one leg in front of you or out to the side, squatting with the other leg until your thigh is parallel with the floor. Come back up, and repeat. Don't forget to perform the exercise for both legs.

SINGLE-LEG CALF RAISE

The last exercise is the single-leg calf raise. This is performed by standing on the ball of your foot on the edge of a raised surface (like a step) and lowering your heel (keeping the rest of your body rigid). Go as far down as you can, then push your body up using the power of your calf muscle. Extend up on the ball of your foot as far as possible. As with the single-leg squat, this exercise needs to be performed for both legs.

These five exercises will give your body good strength and shape stimulation. A repetition is one full movement of an exercise (for example, one repetition of the dip is performed by going all the way down and back up again). A set is a group of nonstop repetitions.

The *Fast Lane to Fitness* freehand workout can be performed in just a few minutes. The more you use this workout (or any workout) the quicker and more efficient your training will become. For example, if it takes you 15 minutes to perform this workout when you begin the *Fast Lane to Fitness* program, eventually you will be able to perform the same workout in 10 to 12 minutes. Aim at reducing the time it takes for you to perform this workout.

The *Fast Lane to Fitness* freehand workout should be performed one or two times a week. In addition to this workout, get in a few sets of crunches for your waist during the week (for example, after you wake up in the morning, or when you have a couple of extra minutes). The *Fast Lane to Fitness* freehand workout should only take a few minutes out of your schedule, yet it will challenge and stimulate your body, increasing your strength and muscle tone. Another great aspect to the freehand workout is that it can be used when you don't have access to a gym or a set of weights. You can also perform the freehand exercises to maintain your sleek, strong and shapely condition.

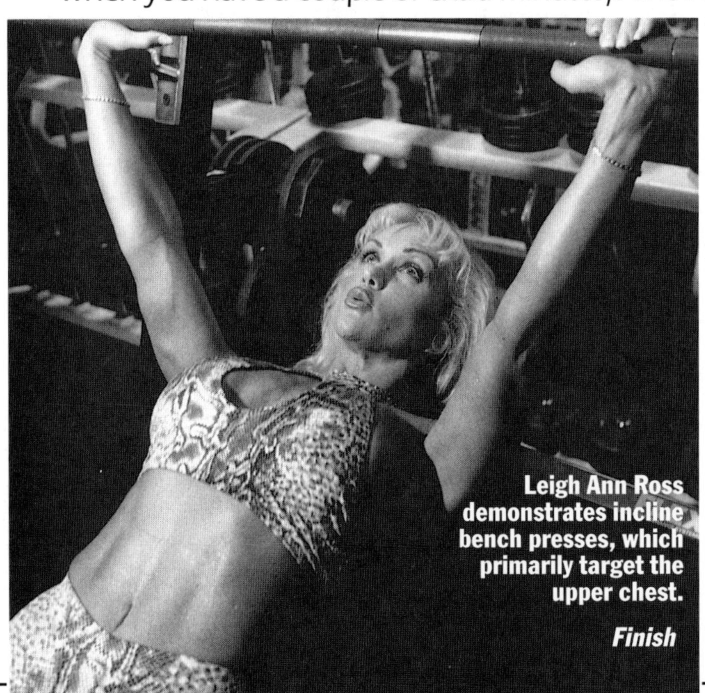

Leigh Ann Ross demonstrates incline bench presses, which primarily target the upper chest.

Finish

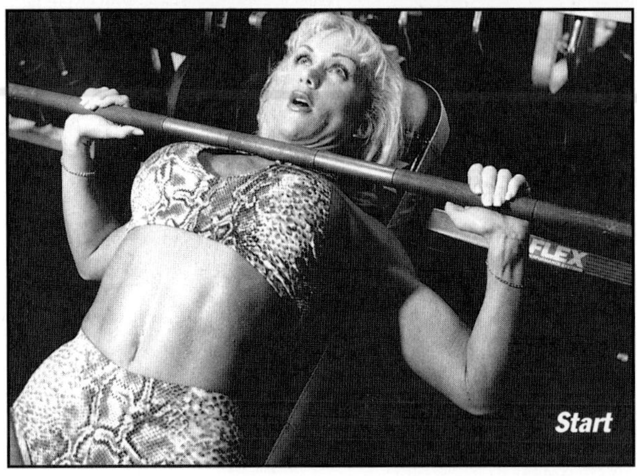

Start

WEIGHT TRAINING

Weight training is the cream of the crop when it comes to strength and shape training. It radically and positively alters the shape of your body. In order to make weight training possible for the *Fast Lane to Fitness* routine, it needs to be brief – brief and effective. To do this it is essential to target the major muscle groups.

BENCH PRESSES

The first exercise in the *Fast Lane to Fitness* weight-training routine is the bench press. The bench press will build the chest, triceps, shoulders, and even partially work the back muscles. It is performed like an upside-down pushup by laying face up on a bench. Lower a light barbell to your chest, then push it straight up to a full-arm extension.

PULLDOWNS

The next exercise is the medium-grip cable pulldown. This movement is similar to the medium-grip chinup. The exercise is performed on a cable-pulley machine. You use an underhand grip (palms up) and instead of pulling your body up, you pull the bar down to your chest area. This is an excellent exercise, working the biceps and the back muscles.

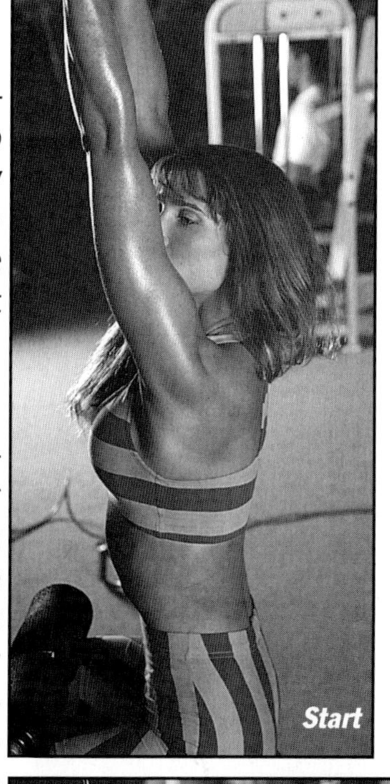

Start

SQUATS

The final exercise in the *Fast Lane to Fitness* program is the squat. The squat is the best exercise for the leg muscles. Fitness star and model Sharon Bruneau uses the squat to shape her awesome looking legs. So does Cory Everson. The squat is performed by placing a light barbell across your shoulders and squatting until your thighs are parallel to the floor. From this point you stand back up again. Put your heels on a slight platform (a stable step or block about two to three inches in height) as you squat. Keep your head up and your back straight.

The bench press is often referred to as the best upper body movement, and the squat is often referred to as the best lower body movement. The *Fast Lane to Fitness* weight-training workout utilizes both of these great exercises, along with the medium-grip cable pulldown. These three exercises really work the major muscle groups of the body, creating an awesome physique. As noted in an earlier chapter, when you increase your muscle tone, your metabolism moves into a higher gear and regularly burns off bodyfat.

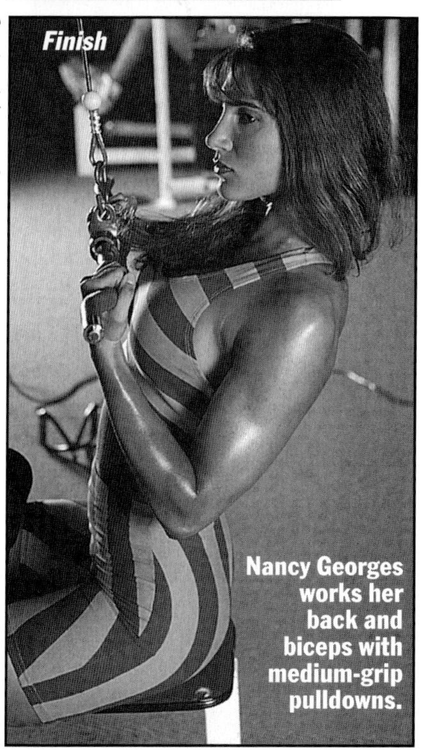

Finish

Nancy Georges works her back and biceps with medium-grip pulldowns.

The more training time you have under your belt, the more efficient and quicker your workouts will become.

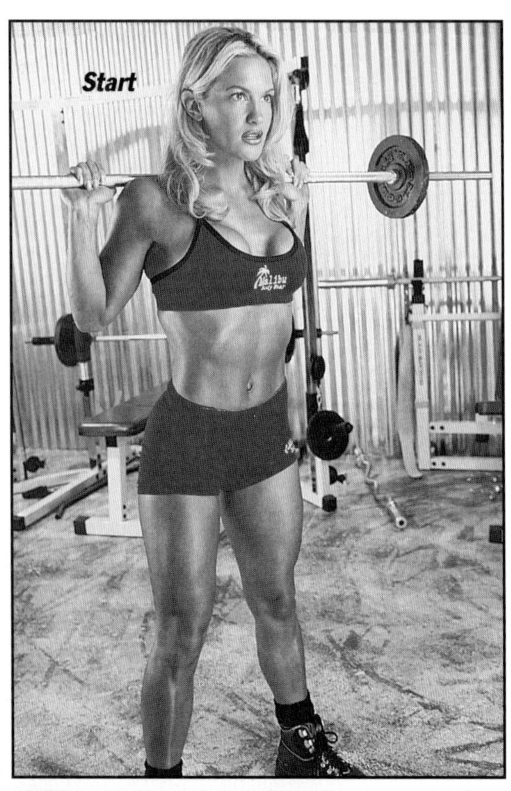

This routine is similar to the one used by Mark Allen, five-time champion of the Hawaii Ironman and 10-time consecutive winner of the Nice Triathlon (the world's most prestigious short-course event). A sidebar from an *Outside* article on Mark noted: "If you're pressed for time, narrow the strength routine down to three core exercises: bench presses, pulldowns, and squats or leg extensions. These work the biggest muscle groups, encompassing 85 percent of the body's muscle mass. If you then find yourself with five more minutes, add abdominal exercises. Ten more minutes? Add dumbell pullovers, curls, and triceps pushdowns." If you have a little extra time you can consider adding the other exercises listed beyond the basic three.

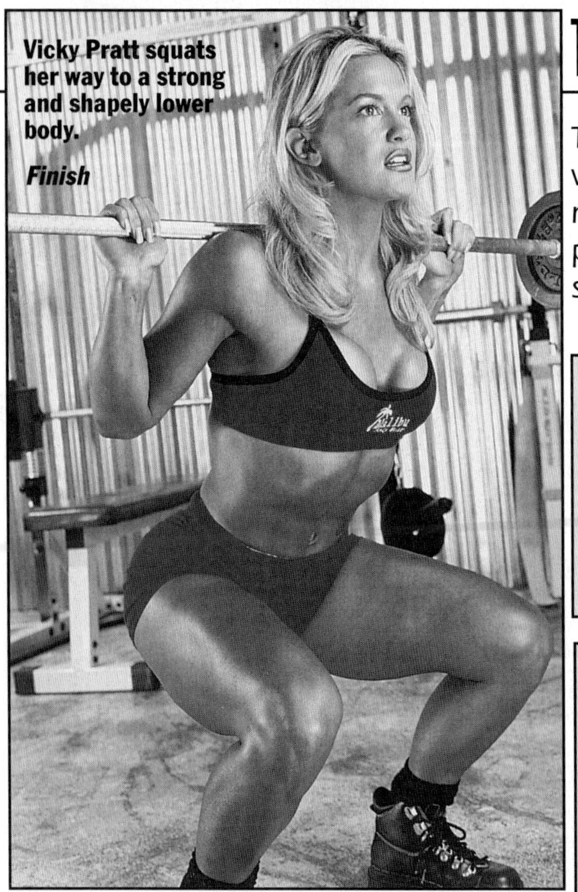

Vicky Pratt squats her way to a strong and shapely lower body.

THE WORKOUTS

The *Fast Lane to Fitness* weight-training workout consists of the three major muscle-group exercises: bench presses, pulldowns, and squats. The suggested set and repetition ranges looks like this:

Fast Lane to Fitness
Freehand-Exercise Workout

Exercise	Sets	Reps
Pushups	2	to failure
Dips	2	to failure
Chins	2	to failure

Fast Lane to Fitness
Weight-Training Workout

Exercise	Sets	Reps
Bench Presses	2	8-15
Pulldowns	2	10-12
Squats	1-2	8-20

As with the freehand workout, you should perform the weight-training workout one or two times a week. (Note – Use the weight-training workout one or two times a week, or the freehand exercises one or two times a week. Your total workouts per week should be a maximum of two.) You can use a weight-training workout first in the week and a freehand workout at the end of the week. If you perform two workouts per week make certain to give your body adequate time for rest and recuperation (at least 48 hours between workouts).

The *Fast Lane to Fitness* weight-training workout consists of just five to six sets. If you are in a real hurry you can perform just one set of each exercise. Make certain to warm up before starting. The full workout can be done in just a few minutes and allows you to condition your body even if you have a very busy weekly schedule. The best manner in which to use the program would be to use it twice a week, but even if you can only use it once a week, do so. Remember, some fitness is better than no fitness. Another factor in your favor is that strength and shaping exercises do not need to be performed as frequently as do aerobic exercises. Your muscles need more rest and recuperation when they are challenged in a strength and shaping manner. Therefore, one or two workouts per week is just fine for stimulating the muscles and giving them enough time to rebuild.

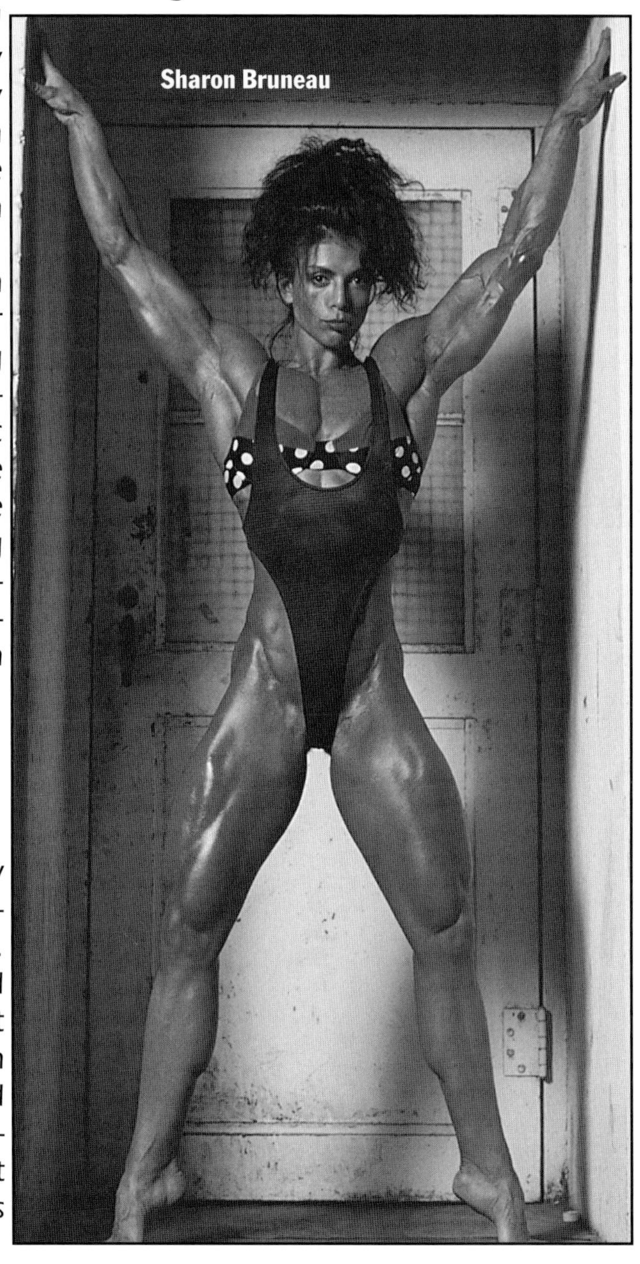

Sharon Bruneau

ESSENTIAL ELEMENTS

There are a few elements – key elements – that make or break successful strength and shape training. These include form, intensity, and concentration. It is very important that you maintain good form throughout your entire strength and shaping workout. Good form promotes good muscle tone. If you start "cheating," by swinging the weights or using momentum to accomplish an exercise, you cheat your body out of the benefits of the exercise. Dorian Yates, six-time Mr. Olympia, uses weight training extensively, and says in *Flex* magazine to "never sacrifice proper exercise form in an effort to hoist more weight." Good form insures that the muscles you want to target are getting full stimulation. An *Ironman* article (February 1996) on fitness star Rene Redden's strength and shape training noted her training is "always slow and controlled." That is the best form with which to work for strength and shape. Good form helps protect against injury.

Hot intensity and good form flow out of solid concentration.

Intensity is another essential element of strength and shape training. Intensity simply means working out at a high level – not just drifting through your workout, but really making your body work on each exercise, on each set, and on each repetition. Intensity means taking your body past the comfort level into the pain zone. The last few repetitions (the last 2 to 3) should be difficult to perform. Instead of stopping when they become difficult, it is important to complete those last couple of tough repetitions. This will insure you are working at an intense level. Intensity helps promote muscle tone. Easy workouts don't change the strength or shape of your physique – only intense workouts do.

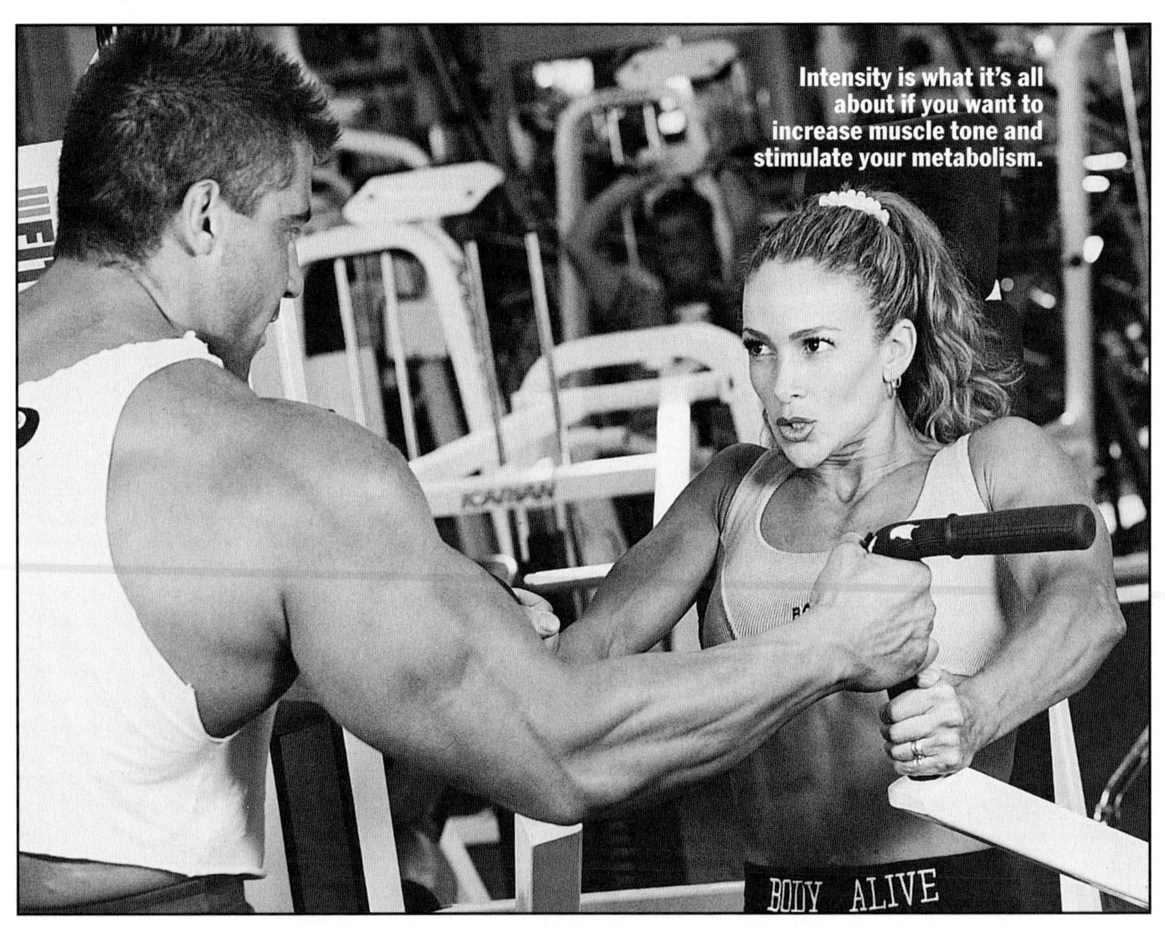

Intensity is what it's all about if you want to increase muscle tone and stimulate your metabolism.

Intensity, good form, and concentration are essential to your workout, allowing you to succeed in your strength- and shape-training goals.

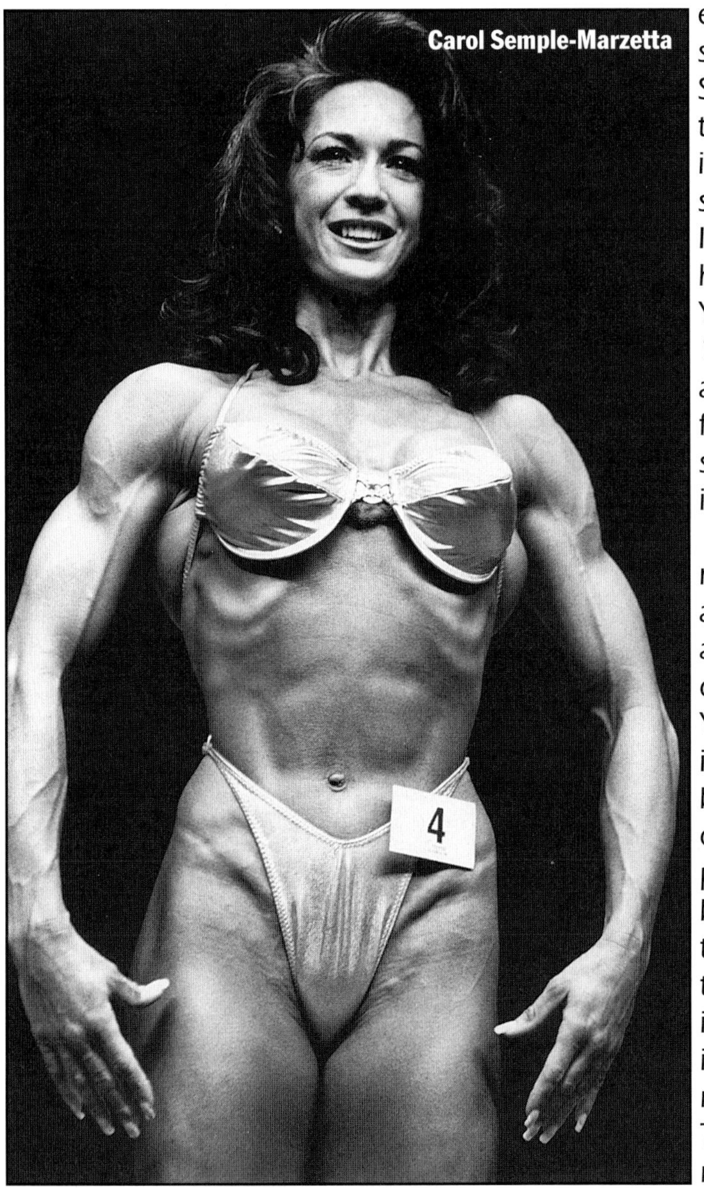
Carol Semple-Marzetta

Strong intensity and solid form go hand in hand with concentration. Concentration is the ability to focus on the workout with 100 percent of your facilities. This means not thinking about dinner, the bills, what you will be doing this weekend, or anything else. Your workout should have your total attention. Since your workout is very short, the time you need to spend in intense concentration is also very short. This makes it easier to achieve. It is possible, and once you learn how to do it, it will become a habit. You will know when you are giving 100 percent. Concentrating during a workout is a very positive, beneficial habit, which only leads to success in strengthening and shaping your physique.

As important as these elements are – good form, intensity, and concentration – they are twice as important for the person who doesn't have alot of time to spare. You simply cannot afford to be lacking in any of these areas. You must bring these elements to each workout. If you do so, you will make progress on your physique that will be evident to all. You do not have to make an extended ordeal out of these elements. Since your workout is short, the use of these elements is brief also. You can gear up internally for a tough workout externally. The key is brevity. It is important to make the most out of the few minutes available for your physique training, and you can do this through intensity, good form, and concentration.

As you train, you will become better at each of these elements. This will allow you more control over your workout, and in turn, more control over your body. Use of these essential inner elements is how you shape and

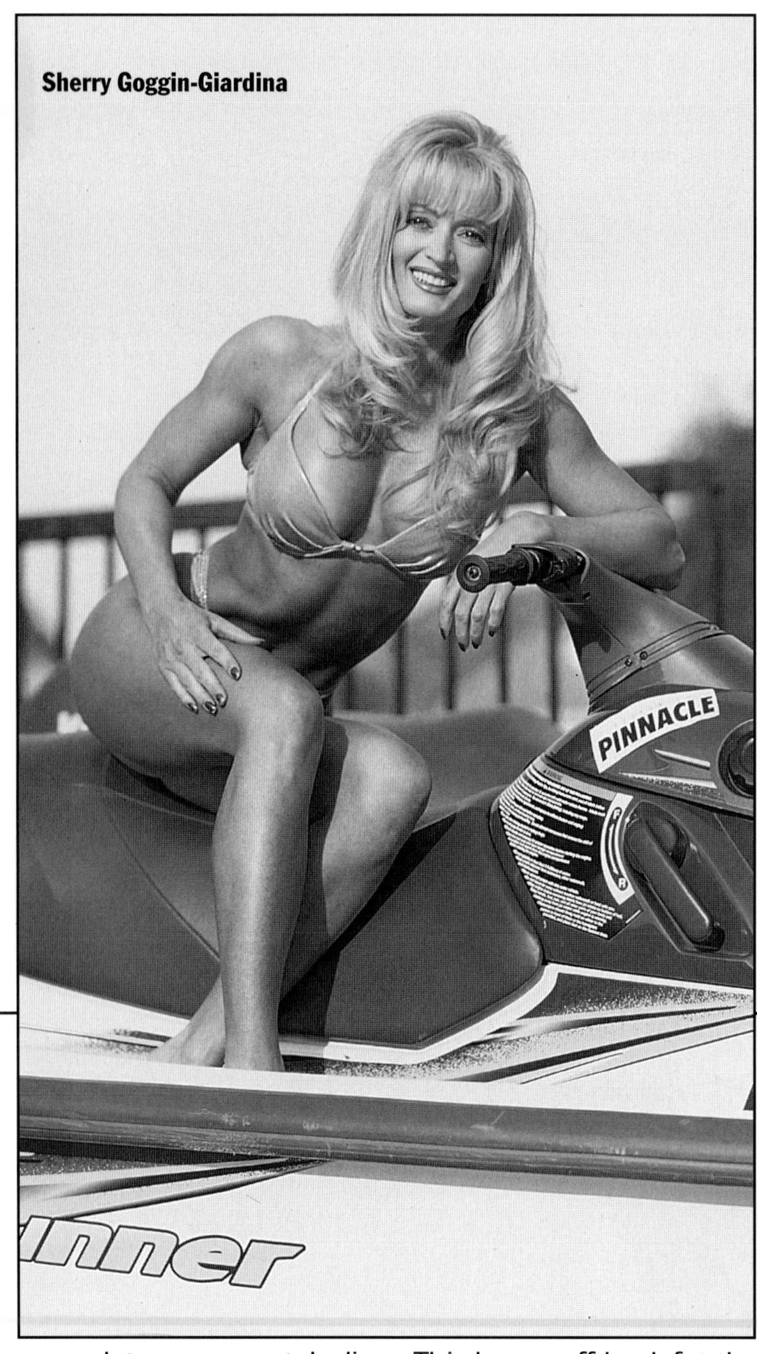

Sherry Goggin-Giardina

Strength and shape training form one of the main pillars of physique training.

strengthen your physique. There is no magic "gadget" or trick to strengthening and shaping your body. The positive changes in muscle tone, strength and shape come from the simple application of intensity, good form, and concentration. If you apply these essential elements to either the freehand exercises or the weight-training exercises on a consistent basis you can build a sleek physique, and do so in a limited amount of time.

PHYSIQUE PILLAR

Strength and shape training is vital to your overall fitness. It greatly increases your muscle tone, your strength, and the positive shape of your physique. It increases your muscle mass, which in turn stimulates your metabolism. This burns off bodyfat throughout the day. Strength and shape training has a multitude of benefits and is one of the main pillars of physique training. It is important to not neglect the strength and shaping aspects of physique training even if you do not have much time available. You can still get in a good workout each week if you use a concentrated routine. *Fast Lane to Fitness* provides a couple of excellent routines (one freehand, the other with weights), which can be used to tone the body in a short amount of time. You can increase your strength and shape on a limited time basis – with the *Fast Lane to Fitness.*

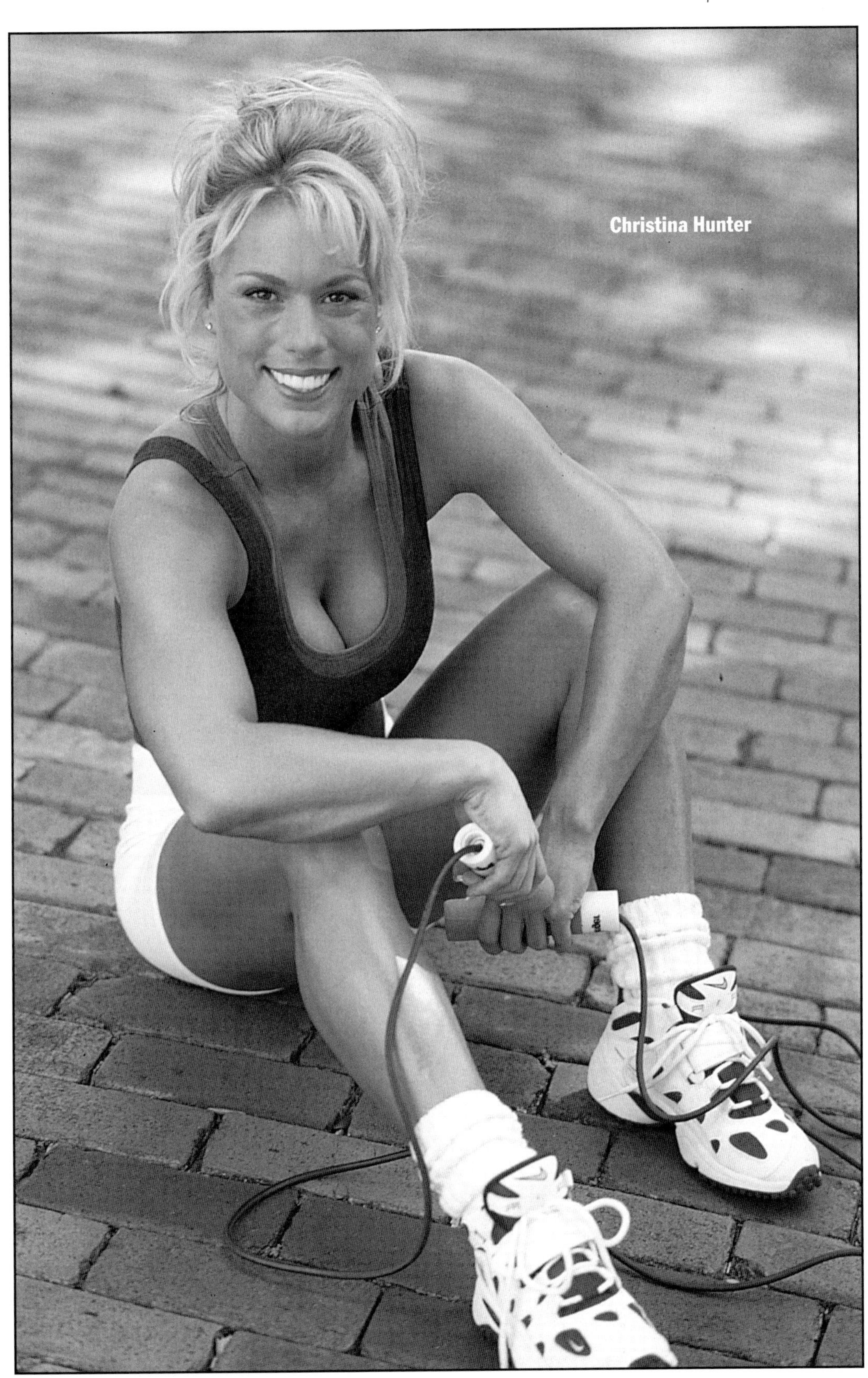

Christina Hunter

Fast Flexibility

Two of the three elements of good fitness have been featured so far in the *Fast Lane to Fitness* program – aerobic fitness, and strength and shape training. The third and final element of the *Fast Lane to Fitness* program is also crucial for your physique – flexibility. In order to take control of your body, you need to have some flexibility training as well. As with the other two elements, it is possible to achieve a good level of flexibility in a short period of time. Flexibility should not be overlooked just because you do not have much time. One of the key factors for success is consistency. You do not need to spend endless amounts of time on flexibility, rather, a short but consistent program works much more effectively.

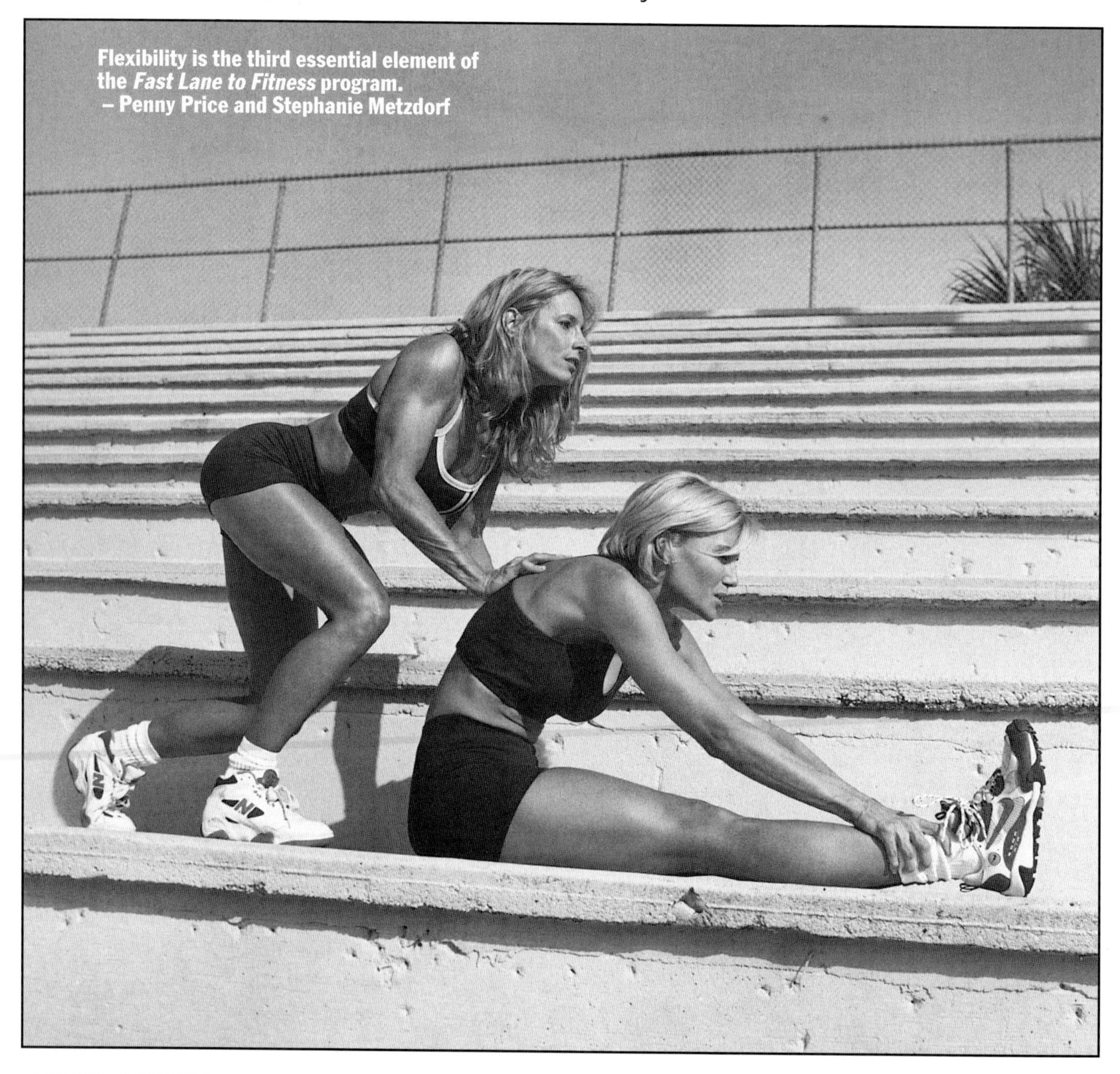

**Flexibility is the third essential element of the *Fast Lane to Fitness* program.
– Penny Price and Stephanie Metzdorf**

WHAT THE STARS SAY

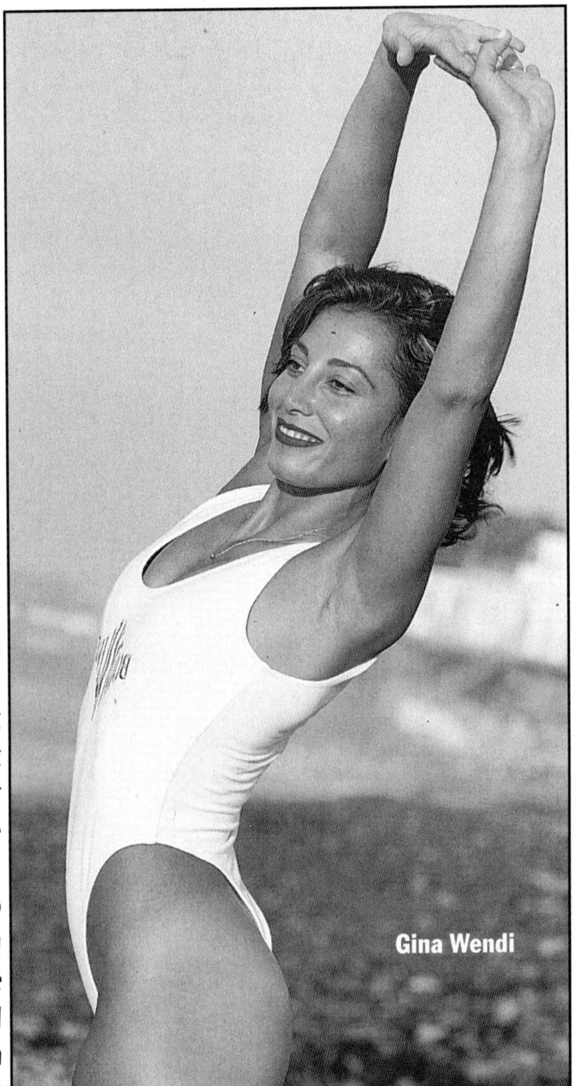

Arnold Schwarzenegger points out the importance of stretching and warming up in his autobiography/ training book: "Very few people have jobs that require much physical exertion. You move a lot without being conscious of your muscles. So when it comes time to exercise, it's important to let your body warm up. You can use that period to tune in mentally as well as physically." As Arnold suggests, the warmup period is a great time to get ready both physically and mentally for the workout. Often you must shift from one environment (home or work) into a totally different environment (the gym). When you take a short amount of time to prepare your body, also use this time to prepare your mind.

For a woman on the go, who needs *Fast Lane to Fitness,* working on the body and the mind at the same time is a very efficient . Arnold further defines the workout time in his book (*Arnold: Education of a Bodybuilder*) by writing, "Give your body a chance to adjust to the new activity. It's a way of saying to the body, 'I'm giving you a warmup now, take your time, fall into it easily. In a few minutes I'm going to hit you hard.' That should be your attitude toward your muscles. Do a warmup of pushups, pulldowns, squats with no weights, circling your arms around and a series of stretching movements. I always warm up the specific bodyparts I want to train." Arnold takes a really light weight and performs several repetitions to get the blood flowing. He uses the warmup to prepare for the heavier lifting, and says the danger of not warming up is that you may tear your muscles and get aches, which will only discourage you from further training.

Gina Wendi

The warmup period is a great time to get ready for the workout – both physically and mentally.

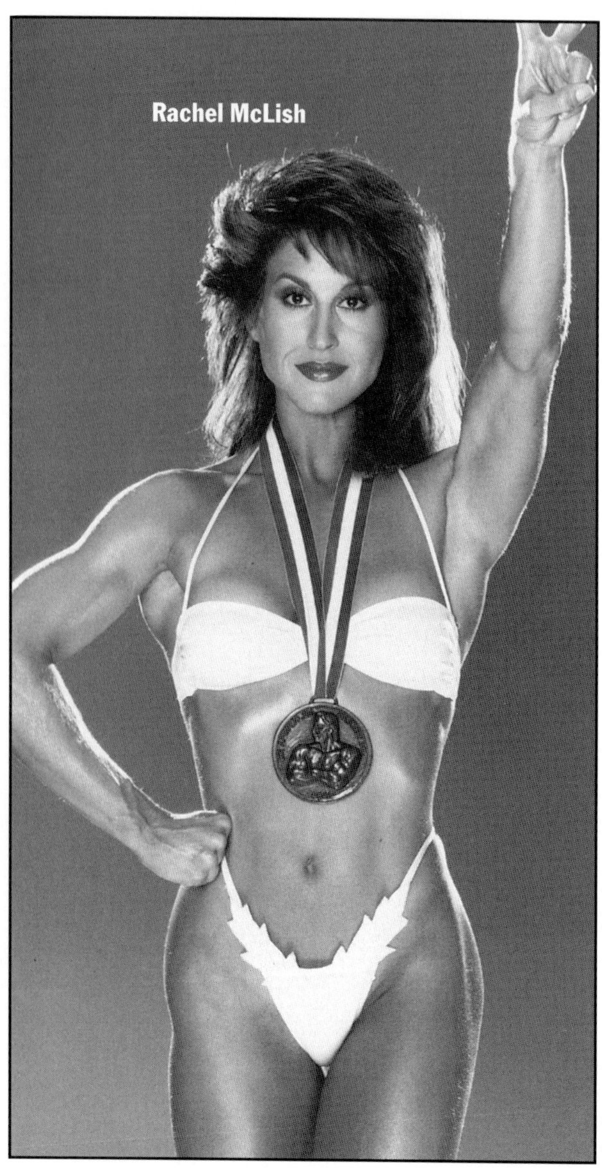

Rachel McLish

Before every workout, prepare your body with a warmup that includes stretching.

If Arnold is considered Mr. Fitness, Rachel McLish has to be considered his counterpart. Rachel was the first Ms. Olympia in 1980, also winning the title for a second time in 1982. She has probably done more for getting women involved in fitness than anyone else. Her books are vastly popular. Rachel believes in warming up as much as Arnold does. She points out in her book *Perfect Parts* that:

A warmup is an exercise or set of exercises that prepares your muscles for the heavy work you expect them to do later . . . a proper workout is just that – it should get your body to a point where it feels slightly warm. This warmth indicates an internal temperature increase in the muscles as a result of increased blood circulation. You warm up simply by moving around – vigorously . . . once you feel warm, perform a prestretch exercise that involves the bodypart you are going to be exercising. This ensures the proper lubrication of the joint(s) there and enables you to work the muscle through a full range of motion. Perform the prestretch before your routine and, ideally, repeat it between each set of reps. The stretching movements send a signal to your brain that opens the neurological pathway, with the result that a greater percentage of the muscle fibers are put into play.

The fitness stars who have made it to the top use stretching as part of their program. Brandi Carrier is one of the elite fitness winners who uses stretching as part of her physique training program. Mia Finnegan and Carol Semple-Marzetta have incredible flexibility and use stretching movements as part of their physique presentation program. Stretching is important and should be given a part in your workout program, even if you don't have a lot of extra time.

Stretching and warmup movements should be performed before your workouts, whether you are doing aerobic work or strength and shaping work. This insures you are flexible and warm. When you work out you are greatly accelerating the rate of many of the body's functions, and putting quite a bit of stress on the frame of your body. It is wise to give the body a little bit of time to prepare for the upcoming workout challenges.

If it is a strength and shaping workout you will be performing, imitate the motions you will be performing but do so without weight and in a slow fashion. Stretch out the area you will be working on. If you are preparing for an aerobic workout, lightly stretch your entire body, especially the legs. Go through some movements that are similar to the ones you will be performing in the workout. Start to get into the workout mentally at this point. Then when your mind and body are ready, go for it!

TWO TYPES OF FLEXIBILITY TRAINING

Fast Lane to Fitness focuses on two types of flexibility – warming up for flexibility before the workout, and a specific flexibility workout apart from the aerobic exercise or strength and shaping workouts. For the benefit of being able to distinguish the two, the first type of flexibility will be referred to as "warmup flexibility," and the second as "flexibility conditioning." Both are essential for first-rate fitness. Both can be done in a short time frame. The first type, the "warmup for the workout" flexibility has already been featured. As

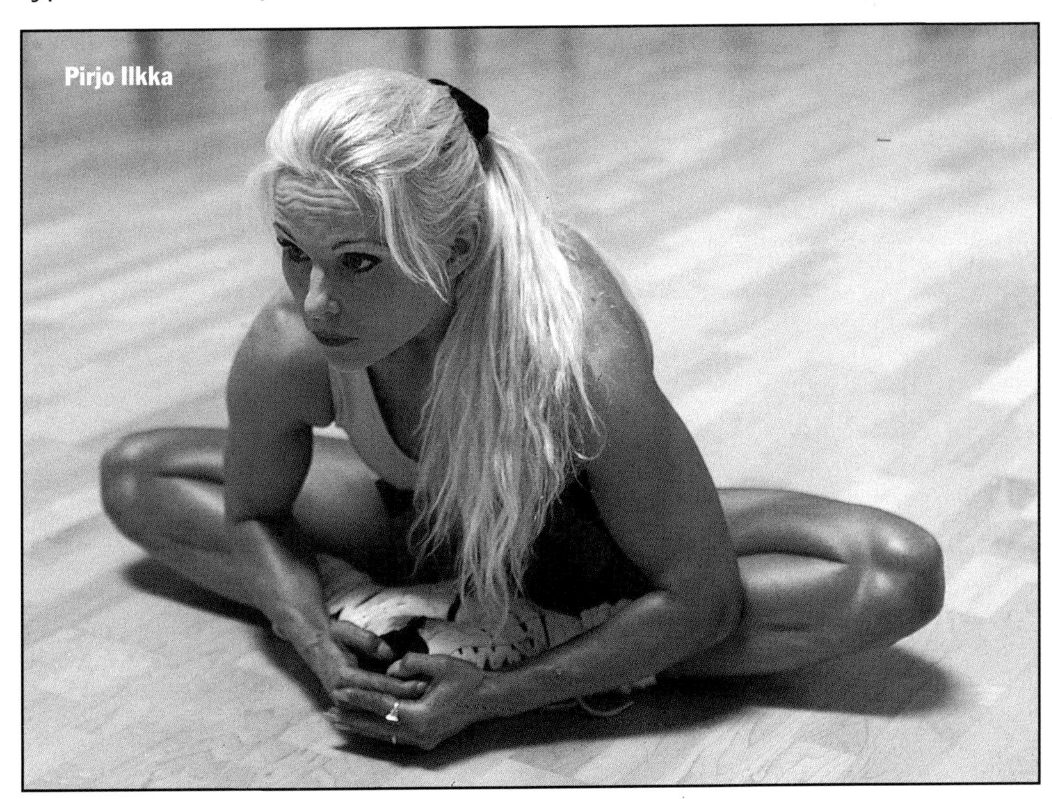
Pirjo Ilkka

mentioned, this type of flexibility involves light "pumping" movements to prepare the body for the workout. The other type of flexibility, "flexibility conditioning," is not necessarily used as preparation for a workout, but rather is a short workout in itself. That is, instead of using this type of flexibility workout as a sidebar to the main workout, it is the center of your workout. With "warmup flexibility" your mind should be focused on the upcoming workout as you slowly increase your physical and mental intensity for the workout. With the second type of flexibility workout, "flexibility conditioning," instead of slowly building up intensity, your aim is to relax.

Relaxation is an important component of flexibility conditioning.

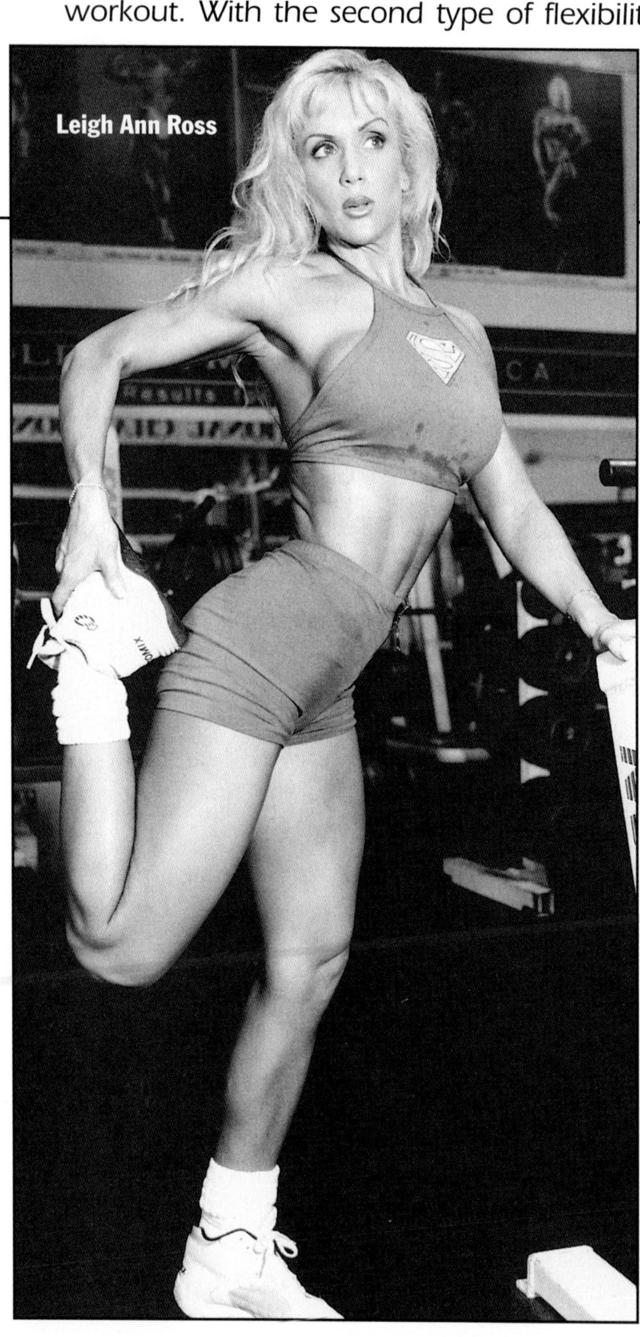
Leigh Ann Ross

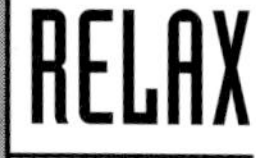

You get the best results from your flexibility workout when you relax. When it comes to flexibility, the best place to look for instruction is martial arts. The martial arts thrive on flexibility. Black-belt holder and instructor Gordon Oster continually reminds his students to "relax." The best flexibility conditioning does not come from tense muscles but from a relaxed body. Martial arts champion James Lew points out in *The Art of Stretching & Kicking* that it is best to "relax into the positions . . . don't force them. Adjust naturally." Lew elaborates, "There are a great many stretching exercises, all of them which have value. Stretching is without a doubt one of the most beneficial, general exercises one can do. It loosens the tightened, knotted, tensed muscles and tendons which inhibit circulation and relaxation . . . keys to success are relaxation and perseverance."

STICK WITH IT

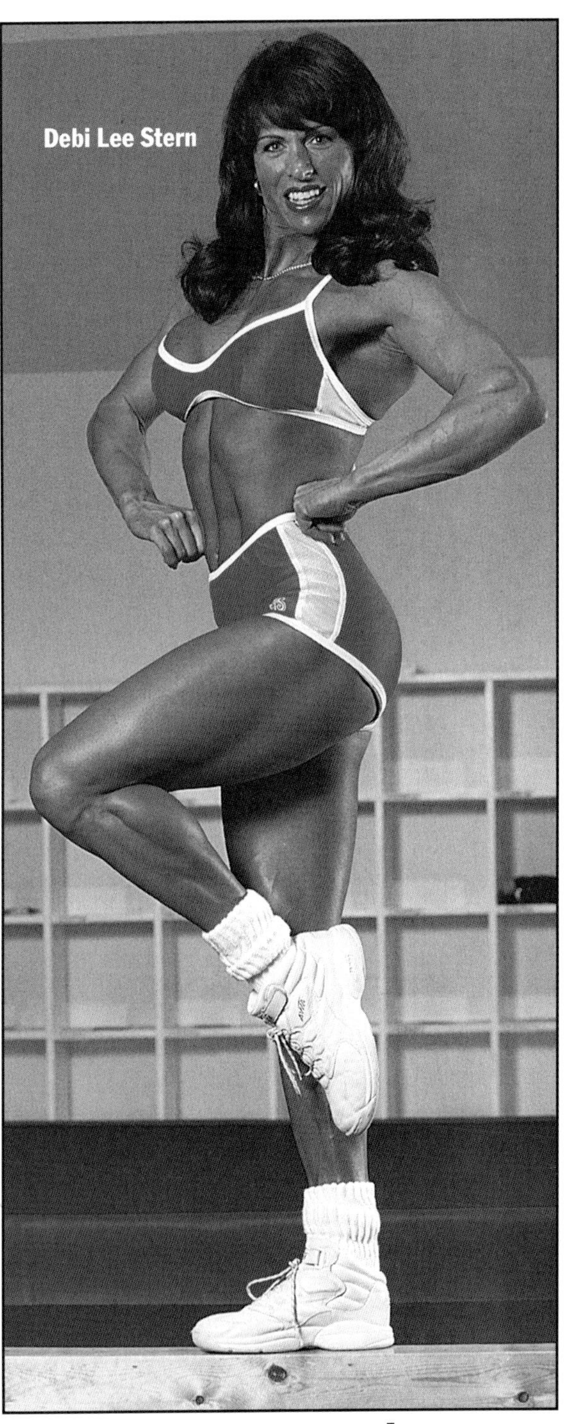
Debi Lee Stern

In addition to relaxation, perseverance is also very important. For aerobic fitness, success is a combination of endurance and perseverance. For strength and shape training, success is a combination of intensity, form, and perseverance. For flexibility, success comes from relaxation and perseverance. The one common denominator is perseverance, (or consistency, as it was referred to earlier). Perseverance is necessary for developing each of the essential elements outlined in *Fast Lane to Fitness*. Few good things happen instantly, yet the "fast" in *Fast Lane to Fitness* refers to the idea that each workout can be short and effective. You will need to perform many short workouts in order to change your physique – in other words, perseverance. You may not have a lot of time in each day, but think of it this way – you do have a lot of days with some time in them. Perseverance will bring about change. This is particularly true with flexibility. As you make your flexibility conditioning workouts a continuous weekly habit you will become more flexible.

Perseverance is a necessary element for success in any type of training – there are no shortcuts to a "hot" physique.

STATIC STRETCHING

The best type of stretching involves slow and deliberate movements, held for several seconds, not fast bursts of action. This type of stretching is called static stretching. Static stretching is the preferred method when performing a flexibility conditioning workout. When you take a position, stretch out slowly and deliberately, remaining there for several seconds. The idea of "remain and relax" is helpful for grasping the concept of static stretching. Don't "dive" into and out of a position. Rather, glide smoothly into the position, and hold it for several seconds. The best way to work on your flexibility is by employing static stretching in your training sessions.

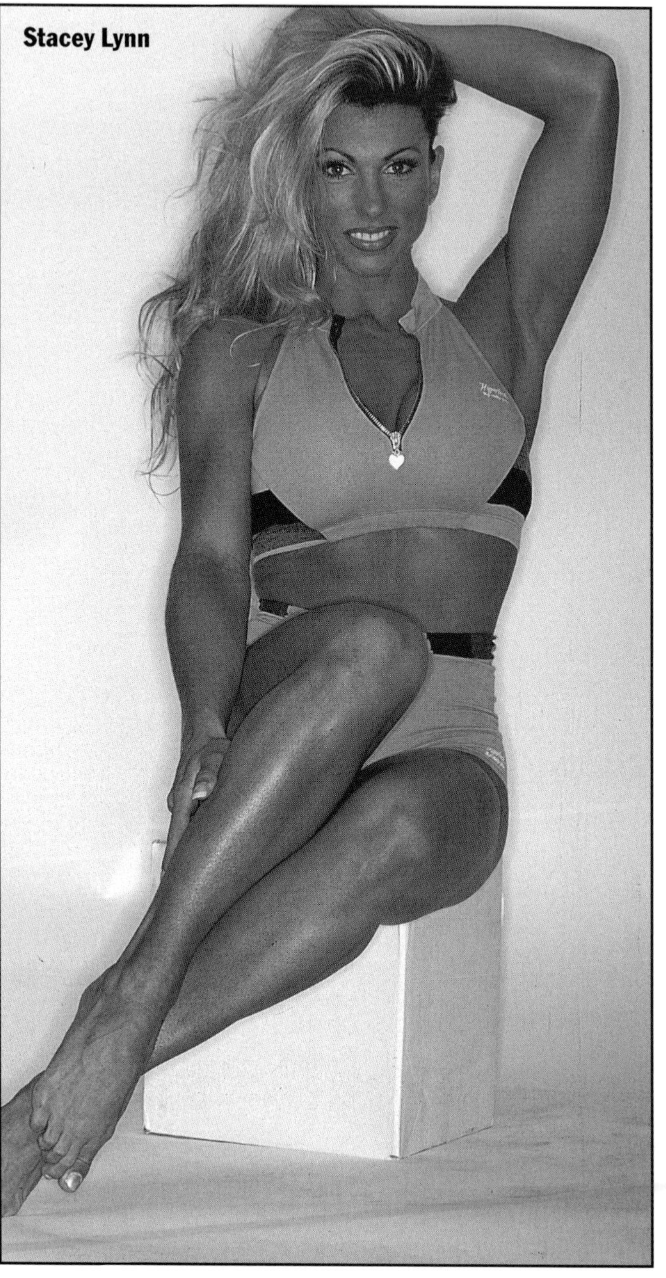
Stacey Lynn

FLEXIBILITY

Now that the importance of flexibility conditioning and the manner in which to approach flexibility training (relaxation and perseverance, and static stretching) have been established, it is time for some specific applications. In order to meet the requirements of this book, the flexibility conditioning workout needs to be basic, brief, and effective. The suggested flexibility conditioning workouts will be broken down into two components – upper-body flexibility and lower-body flexibility. In this manner you can get a better visual picture of the flexibility conditioning routine.

UPPER-BODY FLEXIBILITY

The first part of the upper-body flexibility workout consists of a general stretching session. Stand in an upright position and raise your hands together overhead as far as possible. Hold this position for 5 seconds, then drop your arms slowly out to the sides to form a "T" shape (throughout these movements keep your arms straight, elbows locked). Hold your arms fully extended in the outward position with your palms facing up for 5 seconds, then move them in front of your body and hold this position for 5 seconds. From this position drop your arms back behind you as far as possible while bending forward slightly and hold this position for another 5 seconds. Slowly run through this sequence a couple of times as a start to your stretching routine.

THE DOORWAY STRETCH

The doorway stretch is the first upper-body flexibility movement after the initial warmup sequence. This movement is performed by standing in an open doorway. Put your right arm in a bent-elbow position (forming a 90-degree angle, which looks like the letter "L") against the side of the wall, and slowly step forward with the right foot. Keep the left foot planted in its original position. You will feel a real stretch in the right chest region if you are doing the stretch correctly. To run through the sequence, you stand in the doorway, put your bent arm against the wall, and slowly step forward with the foot on the side of the bent arm while leaving the other foot in its original position. Hold this position for 10 seconds; however, once you have been using the stretching routine for a week or so aim for a 20-second stretch (minimum). Perform the same sequence with the other arm. Perform the "doorway stretch" twice on each side of your body.

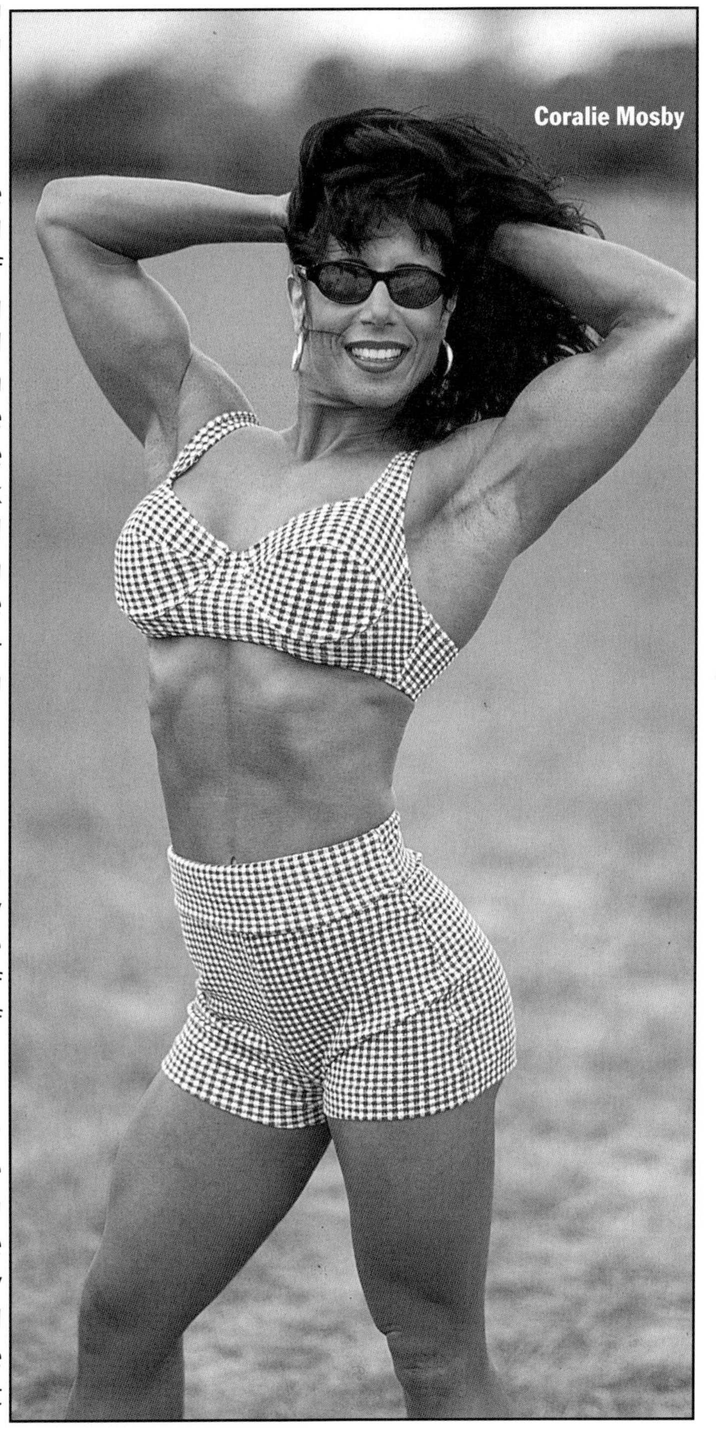

Coralie Mosby

UPPER-BODY LUNGE STRETCH

The upper-body lunge stretch is similar to the doorway stretch except that you are using both arms. Put both of your hands on either side of the doorway above eye level. Your elbows should be bent. Slowly lean forward, letting your body move through the doorway while maintaining your hand position. Use one leg to push yourself slowly forward, then let up and switch to the other leg. Move slowly! Do not make abrupt movements. Start off with a 10-second stretch; gradually increase this over a couple of weeks until your minimum is 20 seconds. Perform this movement twice per workout.

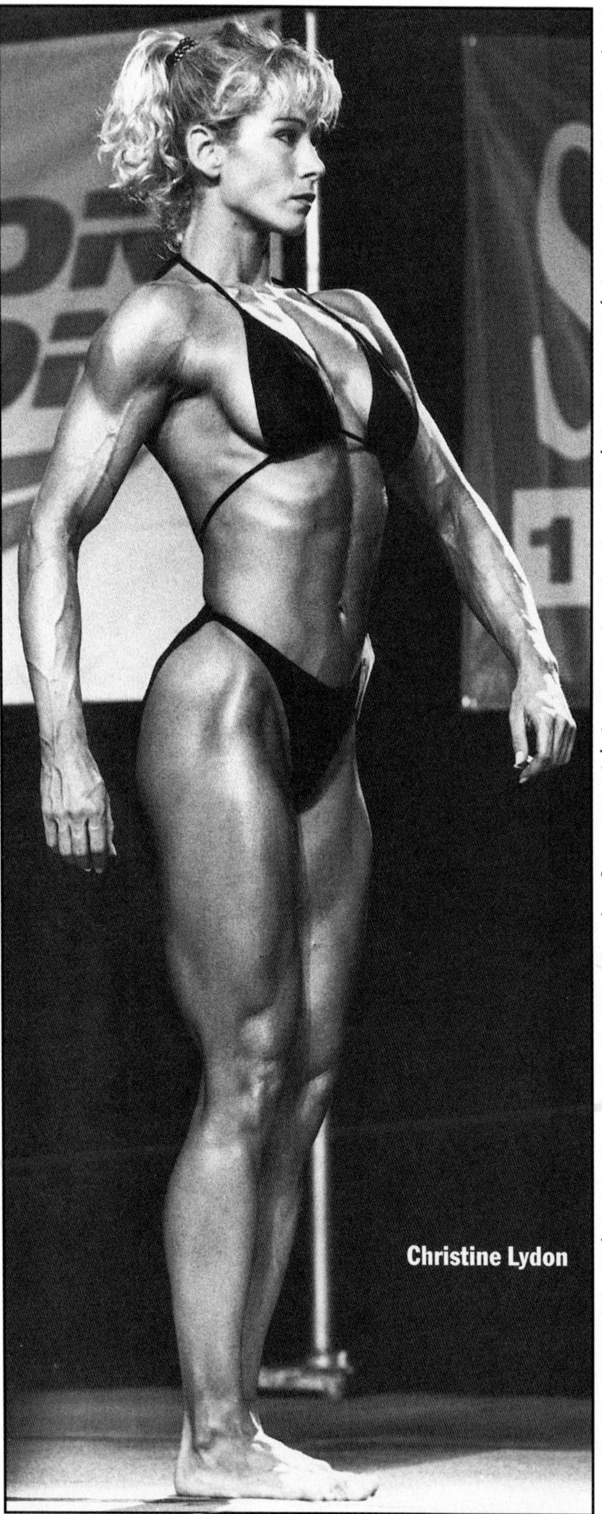
Christine Lydon

BICEPS/BACK STRETCH

The biceps/back stretch is performed by straightening one arm and raising it behind you. Make a fist out of your hand and place the upper part of your hand/fist on a stationary platform behind you (if you are tall, the top of the refrigerator will work; if you are short a tall counter or cabinet will suffice). From this position bend your knees and move your body slowly downward until your trapped arm becomes tight. Hold this position for 10 seconds initially, 20 seconds once you have a few workouts under your belt. If you are performing this movement correctly you will feel it in your biceps and back. Perform the stretch a couple of times for both arms.

TRICEPS WALL STRETCH

The triceps wall stretch is the final upper-body stretching movement (the lower back and midsection are grouped with the leg stretching movements). The triceps wall stretch is almost self-explanatory – you place your arms above your head, (with your face towards the wall) and lean into the wall. This will put pressure on the triceps muscles, giving them a good stretch. Perform the triceps wall stretch twice in each workout, working up to a 20-second stretch.

LOWER-BODY FLEXIBILITY

Most people are more familiar with the various lower-body flexibility movements than the upper-body counterparts. "Touch your toes" is a familiar command from physical education classes. The "hurdler's stretch" is familiar also, as are the splits. For the *Fast Lane to Fitness* program a few will be mentioned – you don't have to know them all.

THE BEND

The bend is performed by standing straight and "touching your toes," or at least attempting to. Always move slowly when stretching. Go down as far as you can. If you cannot touch your toes, go as far as you can, and gradually work up to a point where you can touch your fingers, then your hands, to the floor. Some people who are really flexible may be able to touch their head to their shins. Hold your body in the down position for a few seconds, then come back up. Perform a couple of bends in sequence.

THE SPLIT

The split is performed by extending and lowering both legs outward. You may not be able to go all the way down – so go as far as you can and relax in this position. Stay in this position for 20 seconds or more. Repeat twice.

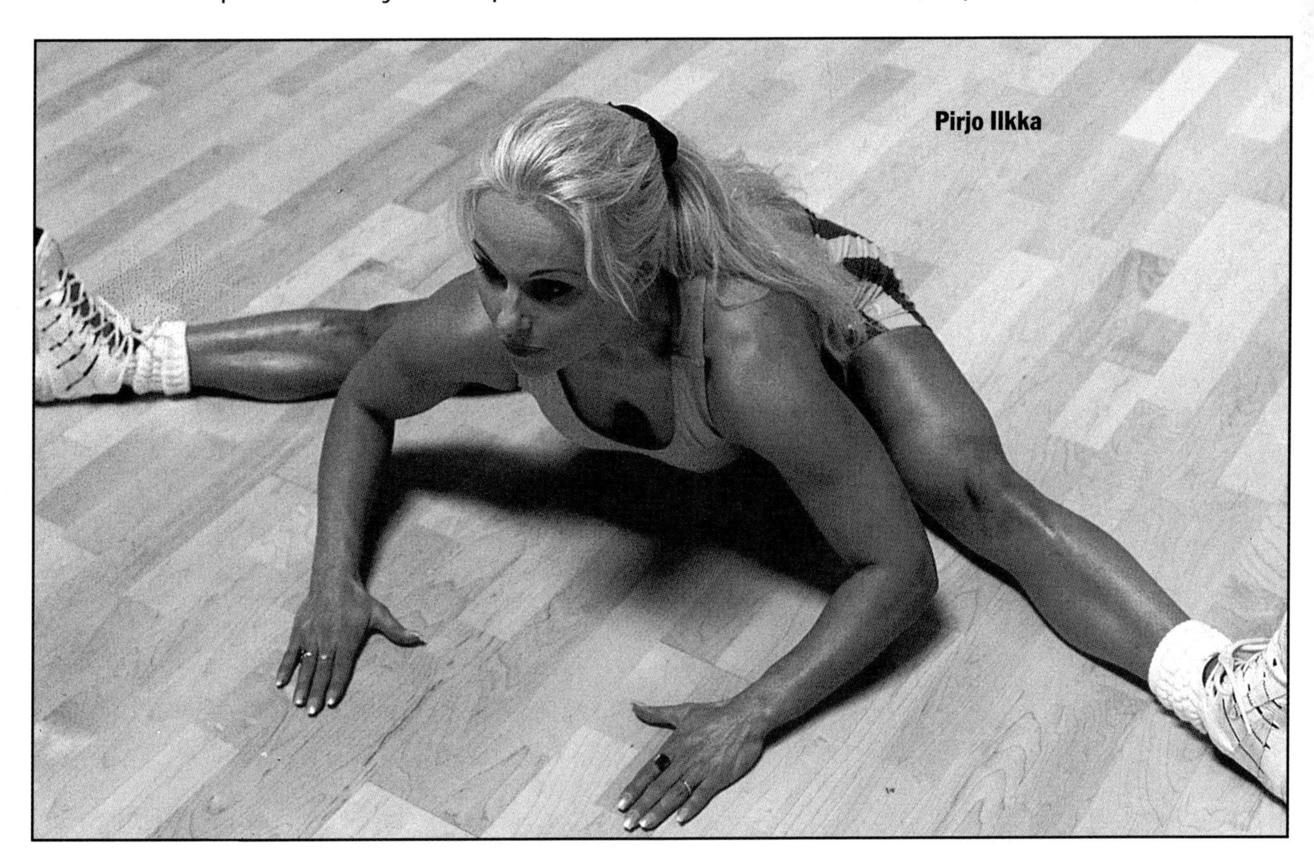

Pirjo Ilkka

THE STAIR STRETCH

The stair stretch is performed by placing one foot on a stair that is at least waist level (you may have to find another stationary object such as a desk to put your foot on if you don't have stairs) and holding this position (leg extended) for 20 seconds or more. Perform a couple of stretches for both legs. Gradually raise the height over the weeks until you can stretch at a substantially higher level than when you first started.

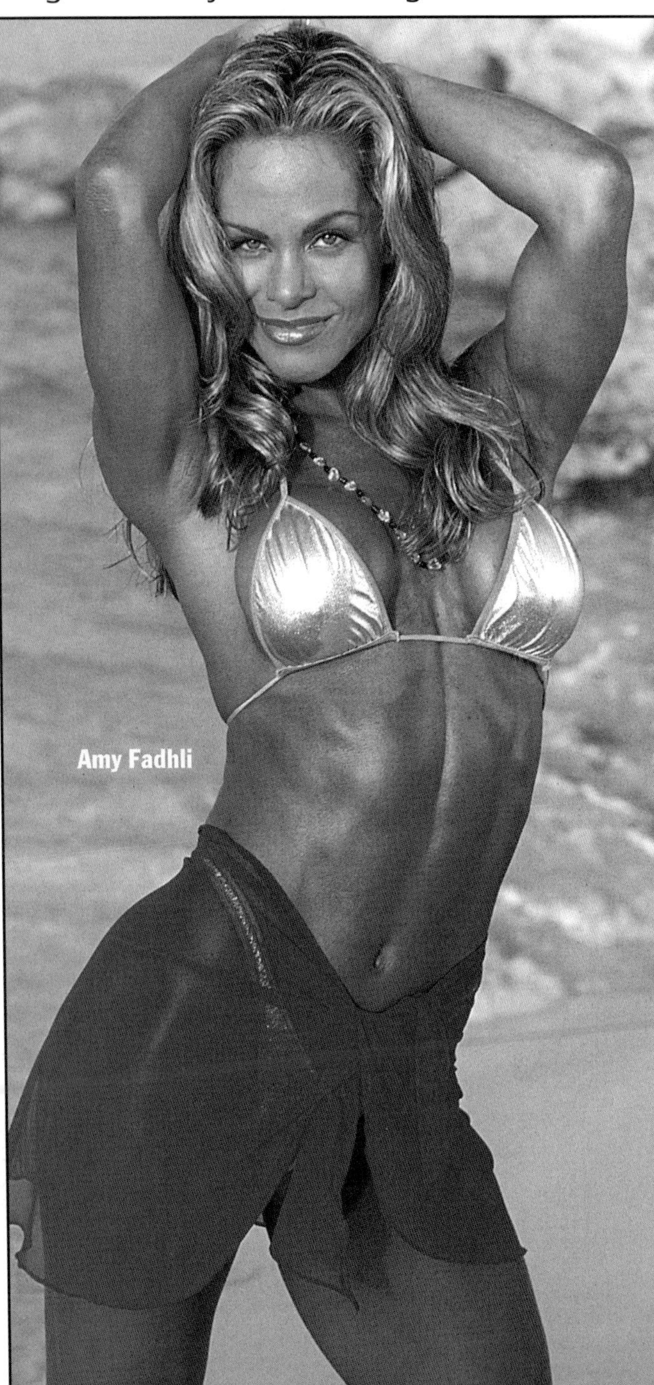

Amy Fadhli

THE HINGE STRETCH

The hinge stretch is performed by placing one foot on a low object like a foot stool or low step and bending slowly forward at the waist. Keep you leg straight and rigid and bend as far forward as possible. Hold this position for 20 seconds or more. Perform a couple of stretches for each leg.

THE TWO-WAY STRETCH

The two-way stretch has been noted by Karen Clippinger in *Shape* (August 1996) as a great way to work on both your calves and your hips: "Stand in a lunge position with your right foot back, and your hands on a wall or post for balance. Keep your left knee slightly bent and the right knee straight but not locked. Your toes should point straight ahead. Slowly shift your bodyweight forward, letting your left knee bend a little more until you feel a stretch in your right calf and the front of your right hip. Focus on keeping your abdominal muscles tight and pressing the bottom (not the top) of the pelvis forward so your lower back doesn't arch. Think about pressing your right heel down and back to fully extend your knee. Hold the stretch for 20 to 30 seconds, concentrating on relaxing and lengthening the calf and hip-flexor muscles. Repeat two to three times on each leg, alternating sides." Notice that Karen points out the importance of relaxing – the common theme in good stretching routines.

THE SNAKE STRETCH

The final stretching exercise is the snake stretch. James Lew describes it in his book on the art of stretching: "Begin on your hands and knees. Push your chest as close to the floor as you can, keeping your head down. Now stretch forward creeping close to the floor. Arch your back as you shift forward, pulling your head back (and up)."

If you don't have a lot of time for flexibility conditioning, cut the number of stretches you perform in half.

The exercises just listed comprise the lower-body flexibility conditioning routine. Along with the upper-body flexibility conditioning exercises, they should be performed at least once a week, and preferably more often. The adage from the other chapters is true for flexibility also – some conditioning is better than no conditioning. If you can only get in one flexibility

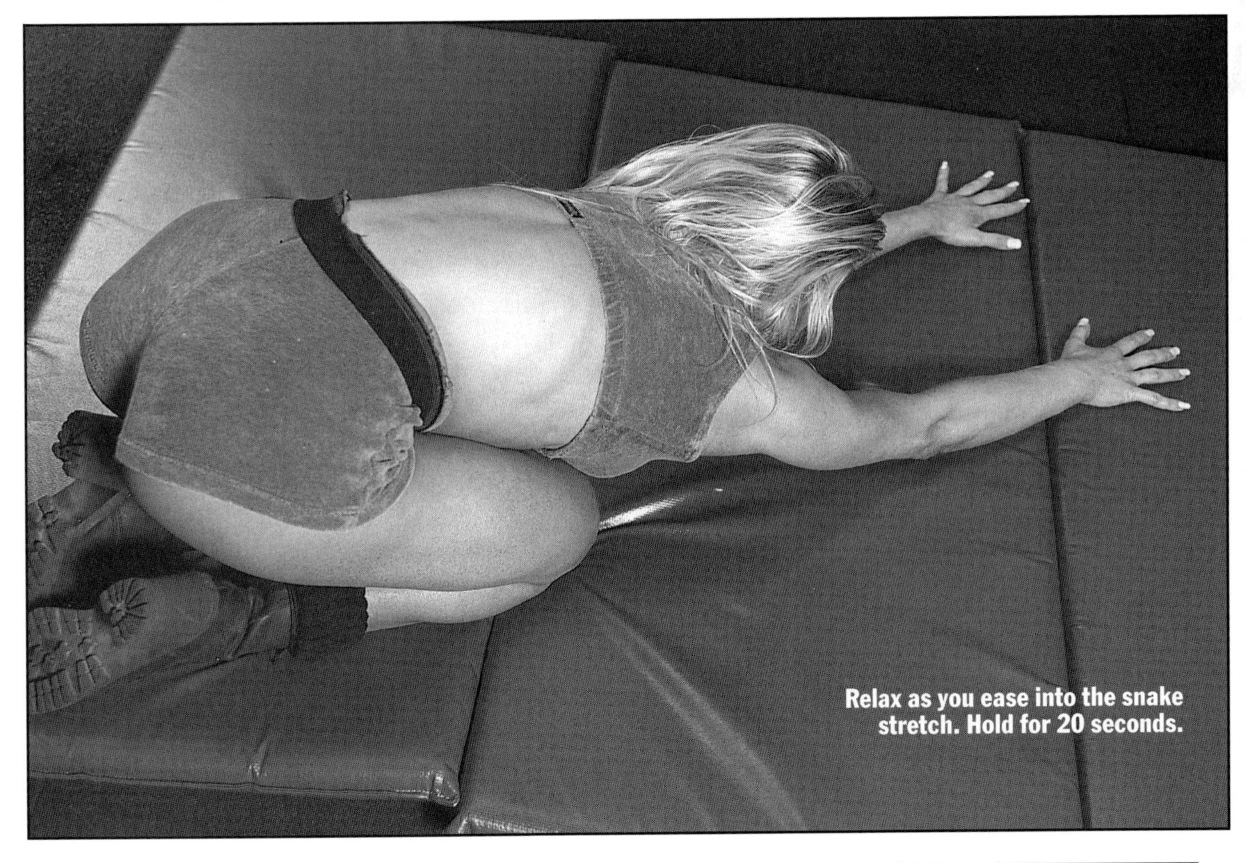

Relax as you ease into the snake stretch. Hold for 20 seconds.

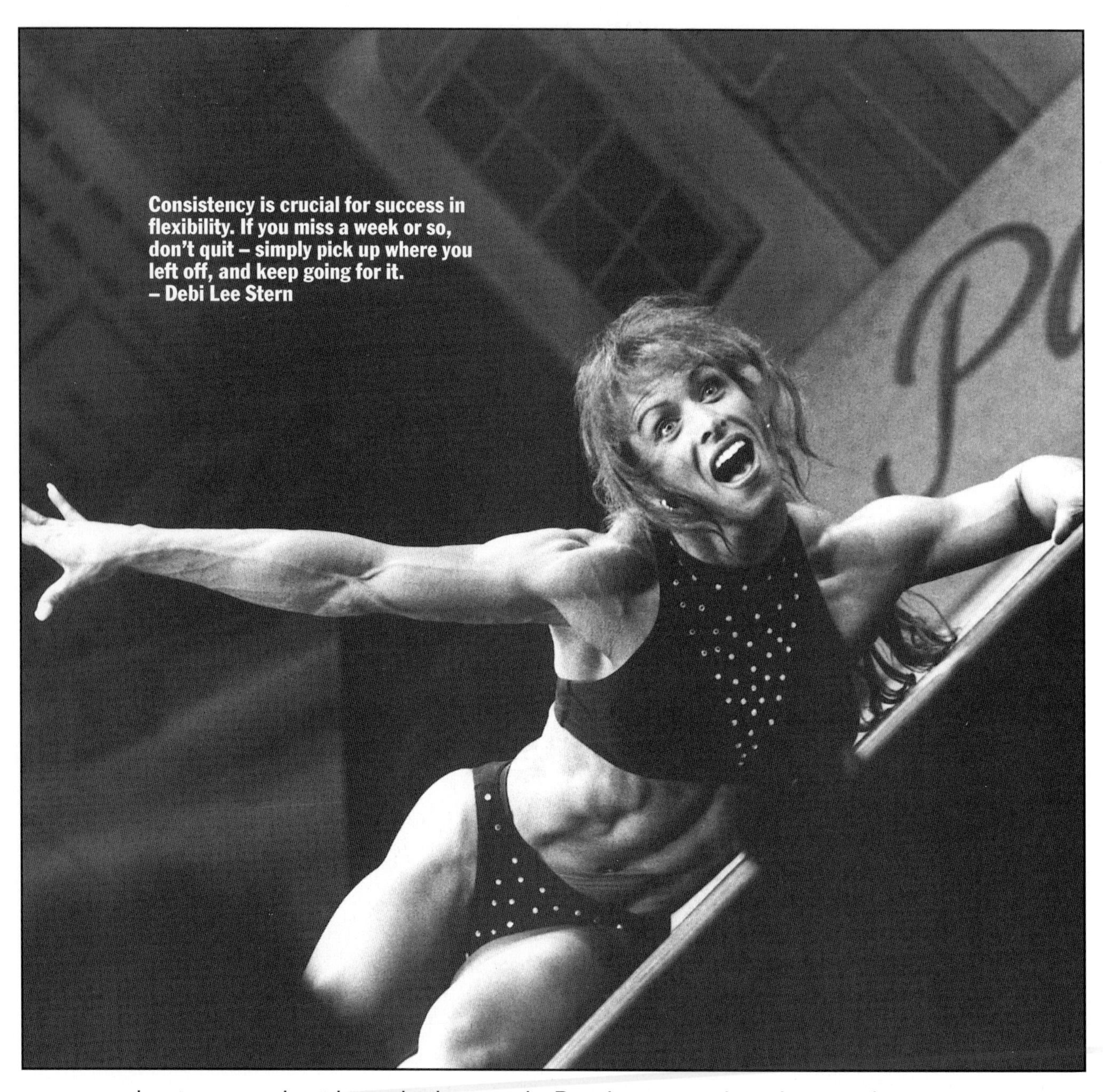

**Consistency is crucial for success in flexibility. If you miss a week or so, don't quit – simply pick up where you left off, and keep going for it.
– Debi Lee Stern**

workout per week, at least do that much. But these exercises do not take up a lot of time and you can get through a flexibility workout fairly quickly. If at all possible, aim at getting in two or three full-body flexibility workouts per week. If you are in a huge rush, cut your flexibility workouts down to a single stretch per bodypart instead of the suggested two. This will cut the time you need for a flexibility conditioning workout in half.

Flexibility is a key component of any good fitness program and one of the three essential elements of *Fast Lane to Fitness*. Flexibility adds a certain grace to your movements. Add flexibility training – flexibility warmups and flexibility conditioning – to your weekly routine for a more supple physique.

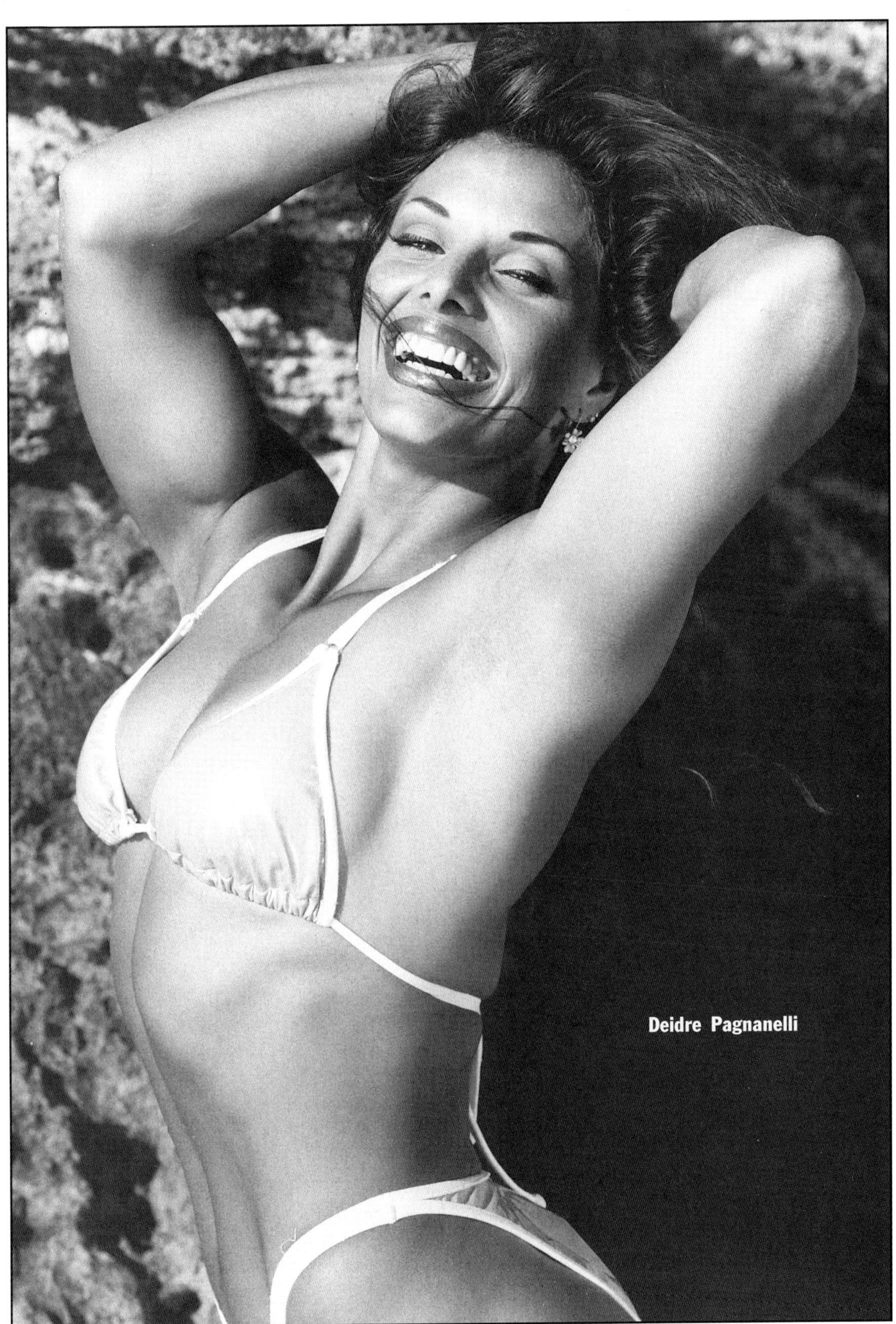

Deidre Pagnanelli

The Quick Mix

The *Fast Lane to Fitness* program consists of three main elements (aerobic conditioning, strength and shape training, and flexibility) which combine to make up a truly balanced fitness program. Balance in training the body (and in the body's responses) should be the goal of anyone who works out. It is not good to neglect any of these areas; conversely, it is important to give each of these aspects of fitness specific attention. For example, fitness competitor Dale Tomita works on flexibility, aerobic training, and strength and shape training all in one week (*Ironman*, February 1997). It has paid off, bringing her national acclaim as a fitness star. Balance in training the body is the key to success. Fitness stars such as April Moore, Marla Duncan, Deidre Pagnanelli, Amy Fadhli and others have a variety of tricks in their bags to control the shape of their body. Fitness is no longer a one-item game. The various elements noted in this book need to be molded together. The trick is in making a fully balanced training routine fit into a busy week. Is it possible? Yes, it definitely is, especially if you have your workout centered on the essential aspects of fitness and have your program organized properly. *Fast Lane to Fitness* has custom-

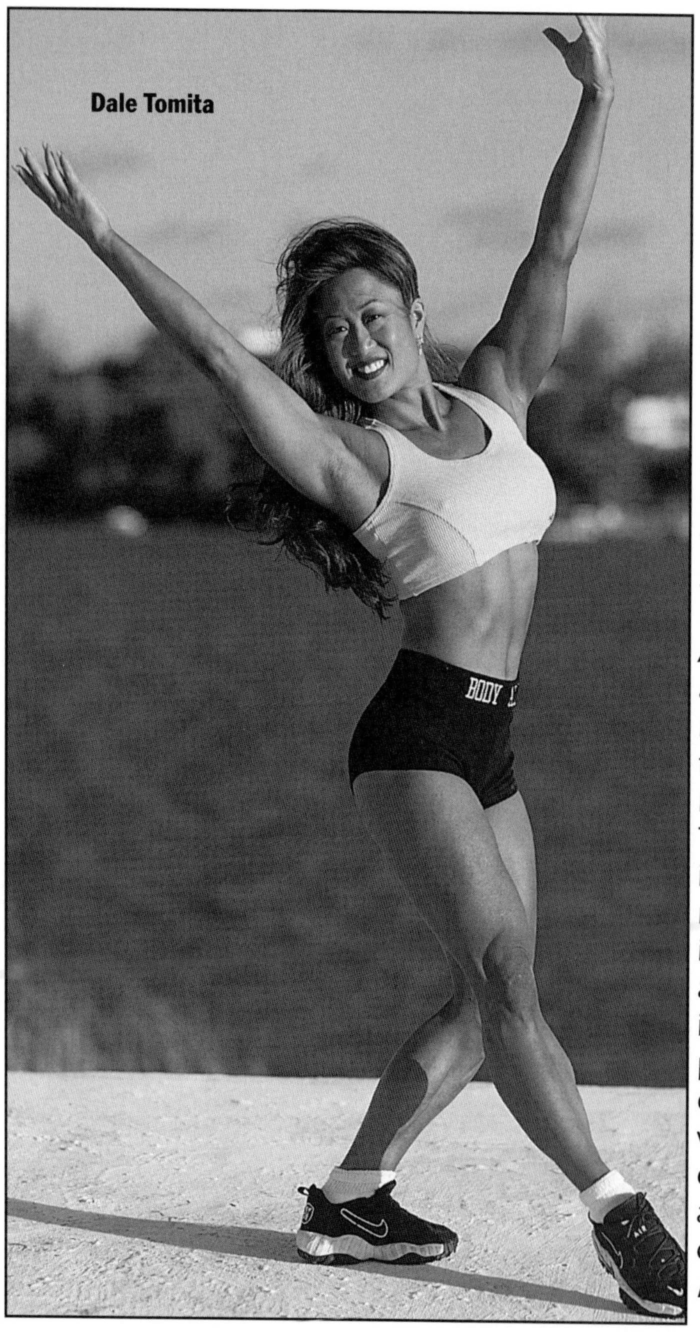
Dale Tomita

tailored each of the three elements into a program that works for the busy woman.

The following *Fast Lane to Fitness* weekly program conditions your body on a weekly basis when you don't have alot of time available due to the daily grind of work and family. Consistency is all that's needed, so add it to the quick mix and you will have a dynamite combination.

WEEKLY PROGRAM

The weekly *Fast Lane to Fitness* program consists of two or three aerobic conditioning workouts, two strength and shaping workouts, and two flexibility workouts. The aerobic component can be any of the exercises mentioned in the chapter on aerobic workouts – the choice is yours. The strength and shape workout can be either the freehand workout or the weight-training workout – whatever you choose. And the flexibility workout can be the one mentioned in the chapter on flexibility, or a flexibility workout of your own construction.

The *Fast Lane to Fitness* program consists of a trimmed down variety of exercises which contain the bare essentials for keeping your body in great condition.

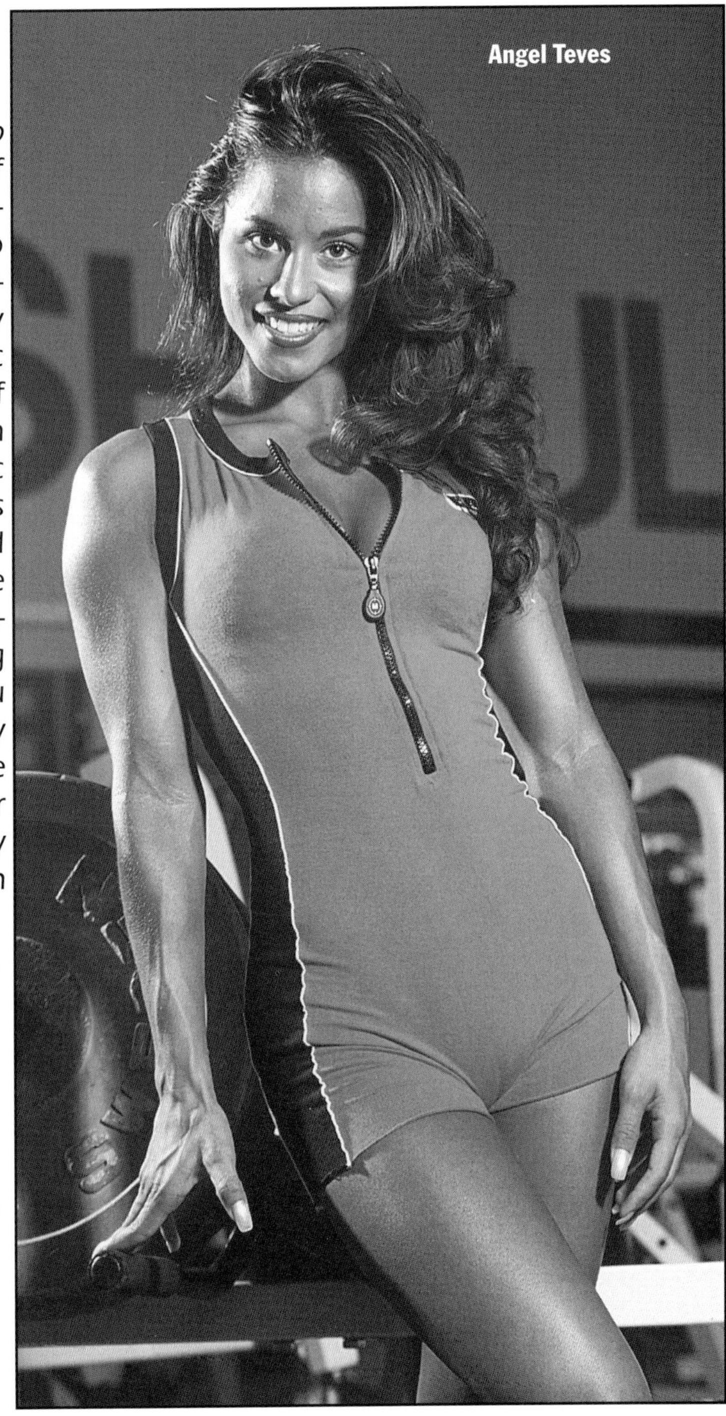
Angel Teves

These workouts should be spaced apart so you have a day or two for rest between workouts. That is, if you perform a strength and shape workout on Monday, you should wait a couple of days (say, until Thursday) to perform another strength and shape workout.

MUTUAL MIX

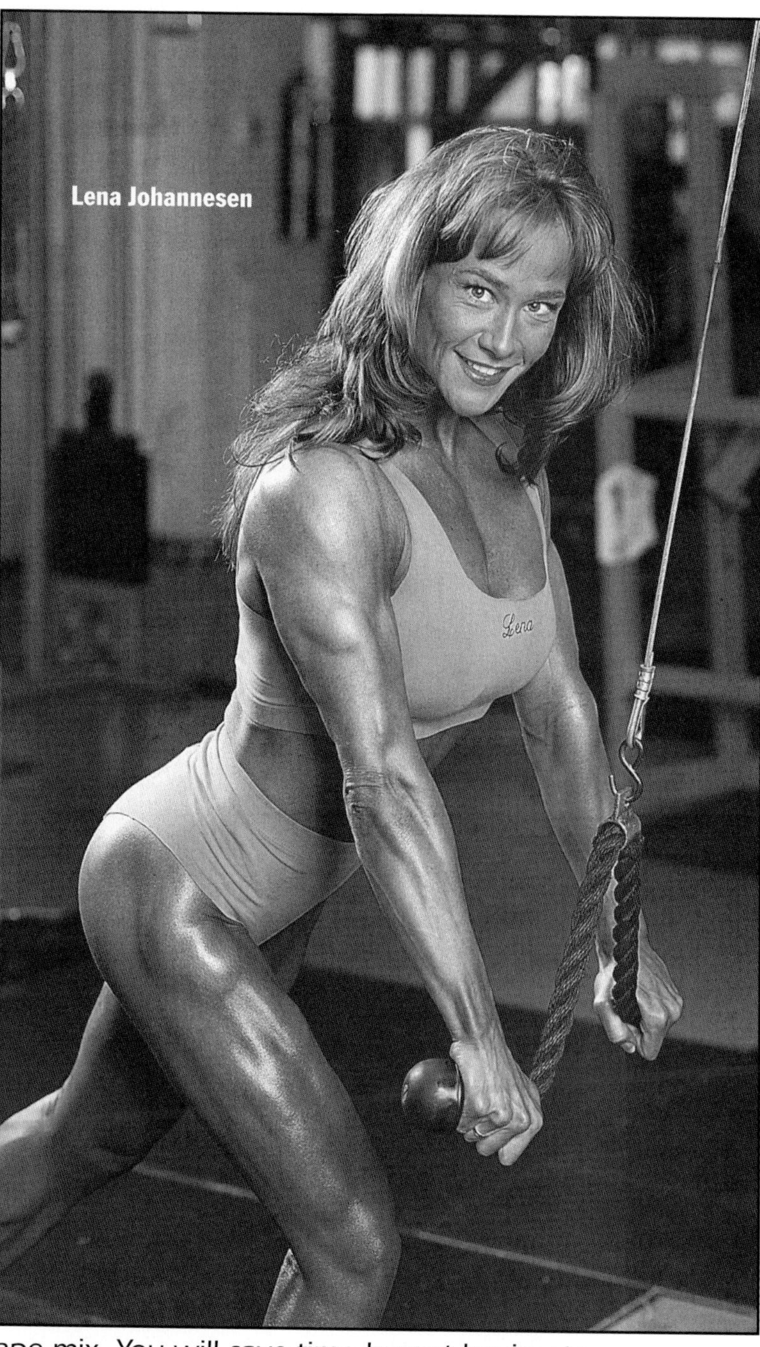
Lena Johannesen

One great way to really take advantage of time, to "double dip," is to mix the different types of workouts together. For instance, start off with a flexibility workout, move into a strength and shaping workout, and finally close with an aerobic workout. This type of set-up provides mutual benefits. By starting with flexibility movements you prepare your body for the intensity of the strength and shaping movements. The intensity of the strength and shaping movements will have your body at a place where it is ready to switch over to use fat as fuel, so that when you do start the aerobic component you will almost immediately start burning bodyfat. Physique trainer Charles Glass points out in *Muscular Development* (March 1996) that it is best to conduct your aerobic work after strength and shape training because "at that time, your body is already prepared to burn fat." There are other mutual benefits with this type of aerobic and strength and shape mix. You will save time by not having to get dressed, showered, and travel to the workout venue again and again – you get it all done in one shot. Since each of the three individual parts of the workout are short, the entire three-part routine is capable of being performed in a very short time frame.

The general *Fast Lane to Fitness* mix consists of two full workouts (combining flexibility, strength and shaping, and aerobics) and an additional third aerobic workout if possible.

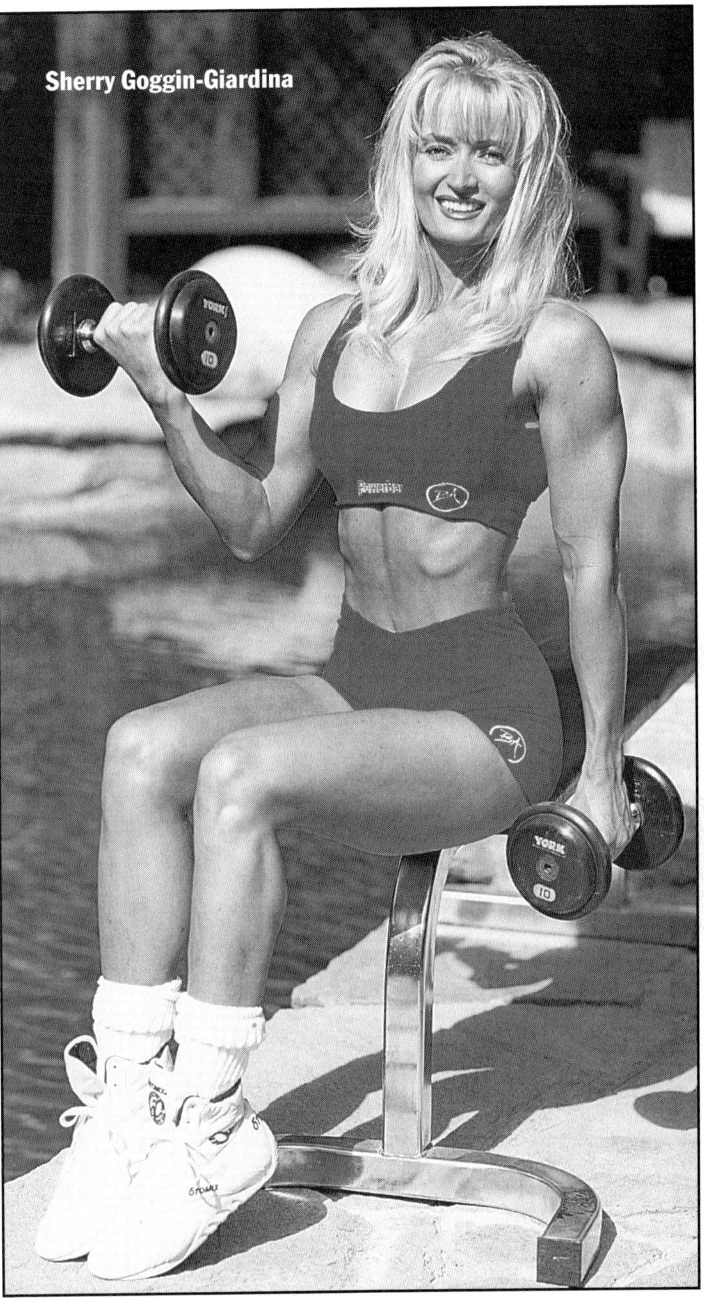

Sherry Goggin-Giardina

THE SUPER SHORT ROUTINE

Some people need a weekly routine that is even briefer than the *Fast Lane to Fitness* weekly program, which includes a couple of rotations through each of the three elements. The super short routine consists of a very brief weekly workout schedule – one flexibility workout, one strength and shaping workout, and one or two aerobic workouts. Additionally, cut the amount of sets per exercise down to one for both the strength and shaping routine and the flexibility routine.

TRAINING TIME TIPS

There are a couple of other tips for making the *Fast Lane to Fitness* training routine work for you. Perform your flexibility movements in either the morning or evening, just as you get up or right before you go to bed. This will leave you more time throughout the day to work on the other two aspects of fitness. Another idea is to use time in front of the television for getting in an aerobic workout. Lunch and break times are also prime opportunities to work on your physique – get in a run or power walk. You'll be charged for the day and ready to tackle anything once you get back to work.

Consistent exercise is the most effective manner in which to significantly change the physique.

AIM AT CONSISTENCY

Whether your fitness routine will work or not comes down to consistency. The importance of consistency cannot be stressed enough. Physique champion Lenda Murray points out in *Flex* (January 1996) that "it requires patience . . . give yourself time."

Even if you can only get in one workout a week, do it! If you miss a week or two – don't quit – simply get started again. Your body won't become conditioned automatically – you have to work at it. The best way to condition and tone your body is through consistent exercise. You don't need any "super" routine or some plastic "gimmick" that is sold on television. You just need to work out with the three main elements of fitness (aerobic, strength and shape, and flexibility) on a consistent basis. You don't have to use a lot of time per week to do so. A couple of good workouts per week will have a significant impact on your physique. Even one is better than nothing. So don't give up on your body even if you don't have a lot of time available to work out. Remember the motto that "some fitness is better than no fitness." Use the guidelines and conditioning programs in *Fast Lane to Fitness* to your advantage and build a sleek physique in a limited amount of time. Go for it!

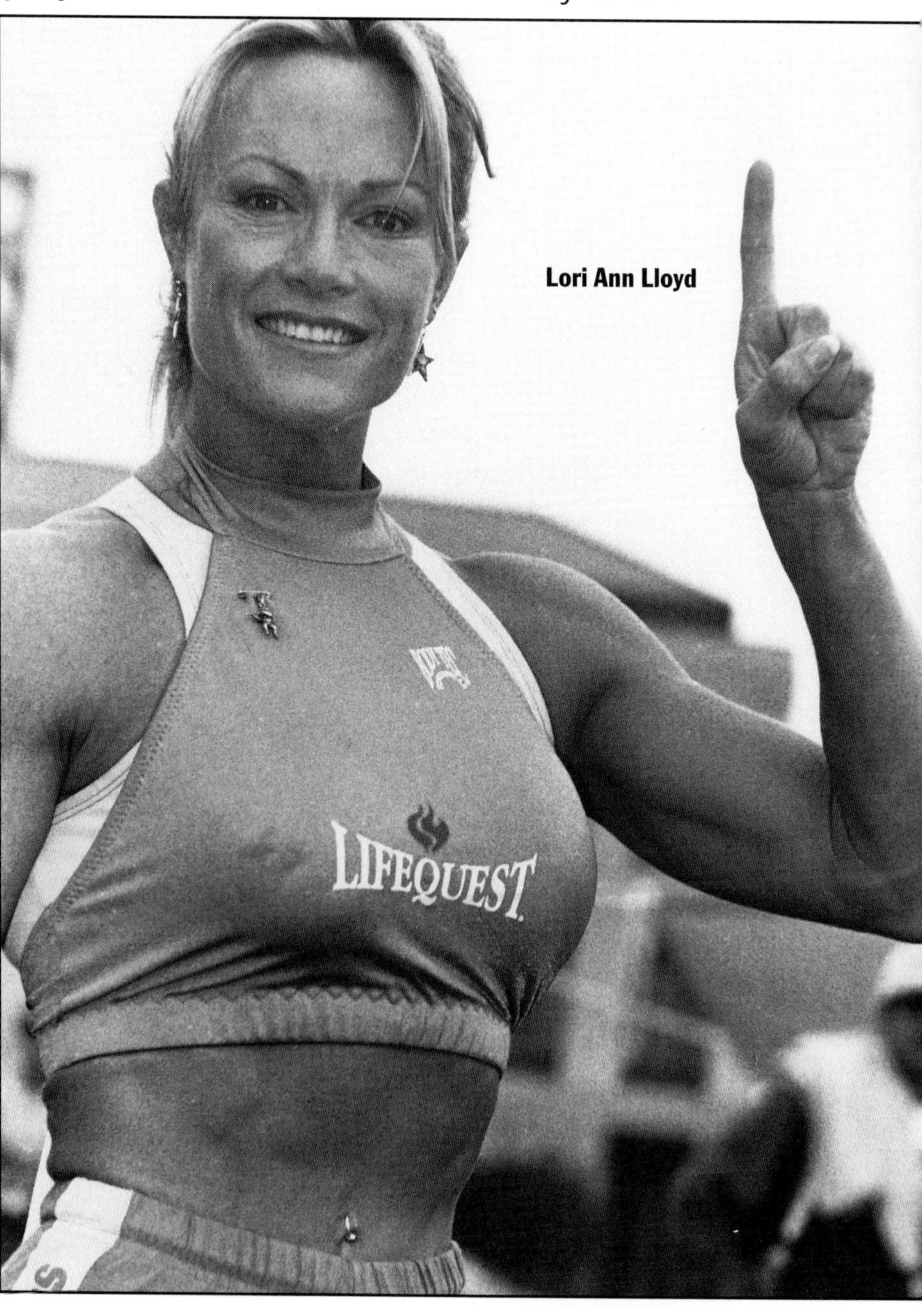

Lori Ann Lloyd

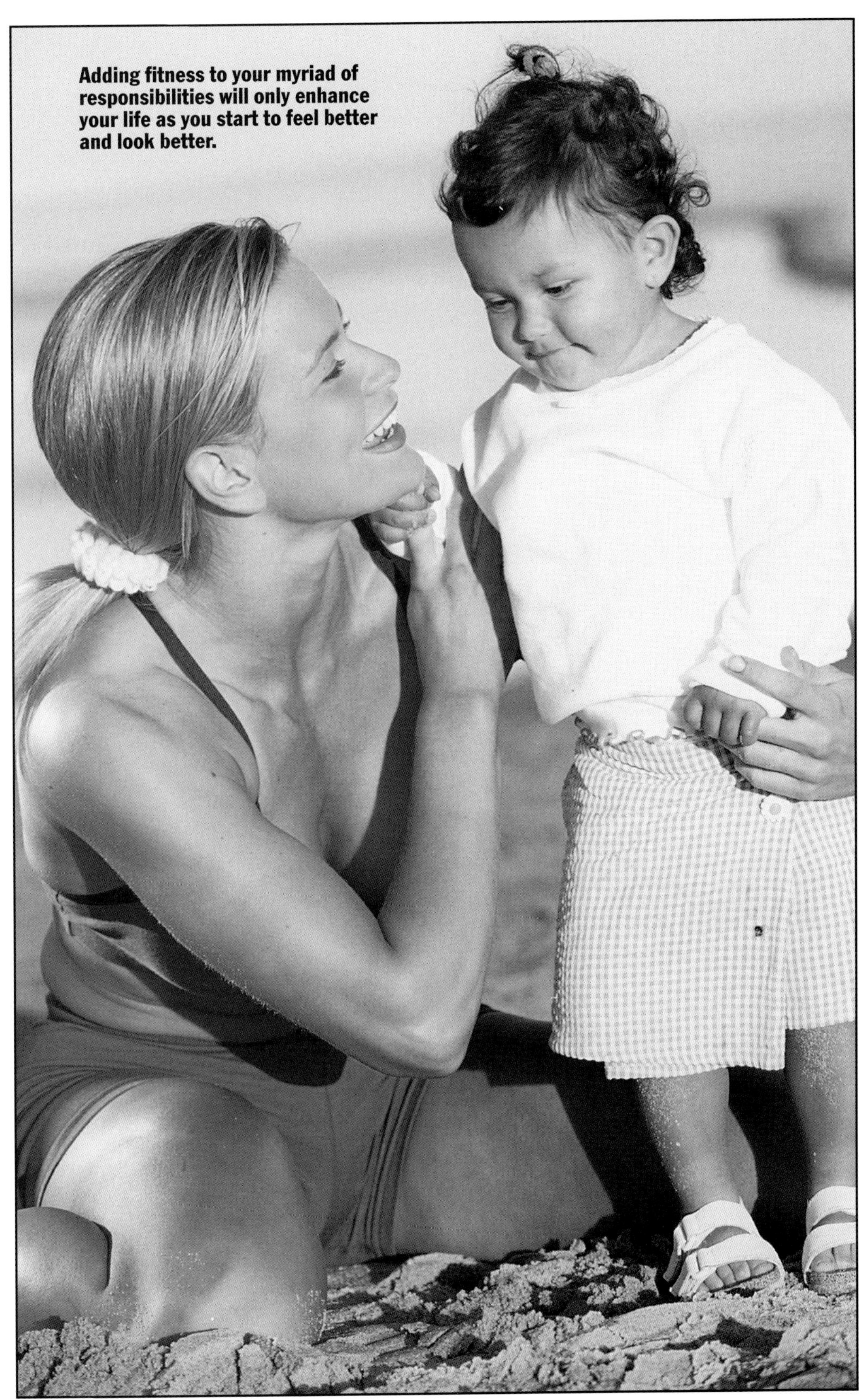
Adding fitness to your myriad of responsibilities will only enhance your life as you start to feel better and look better.

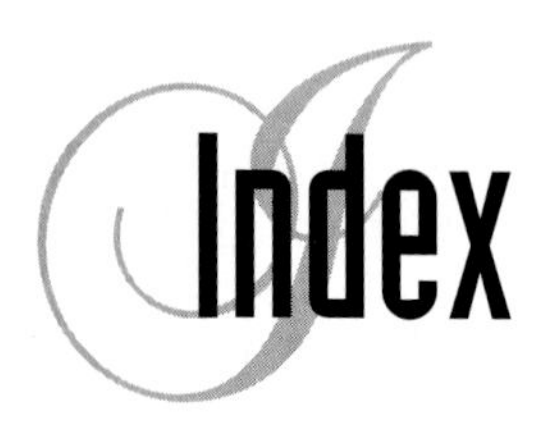

Index

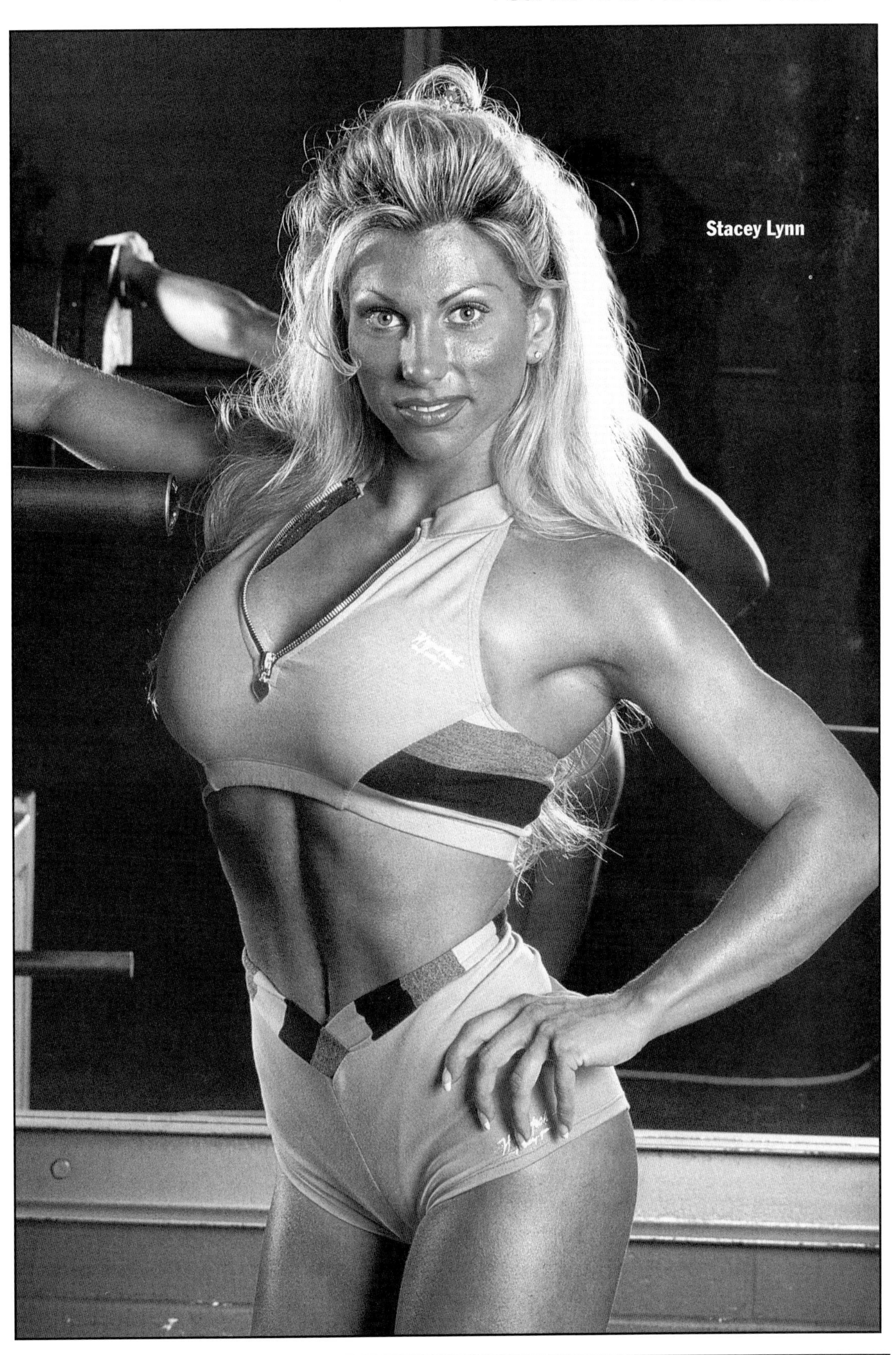

Stacey Lynn

Photo Index

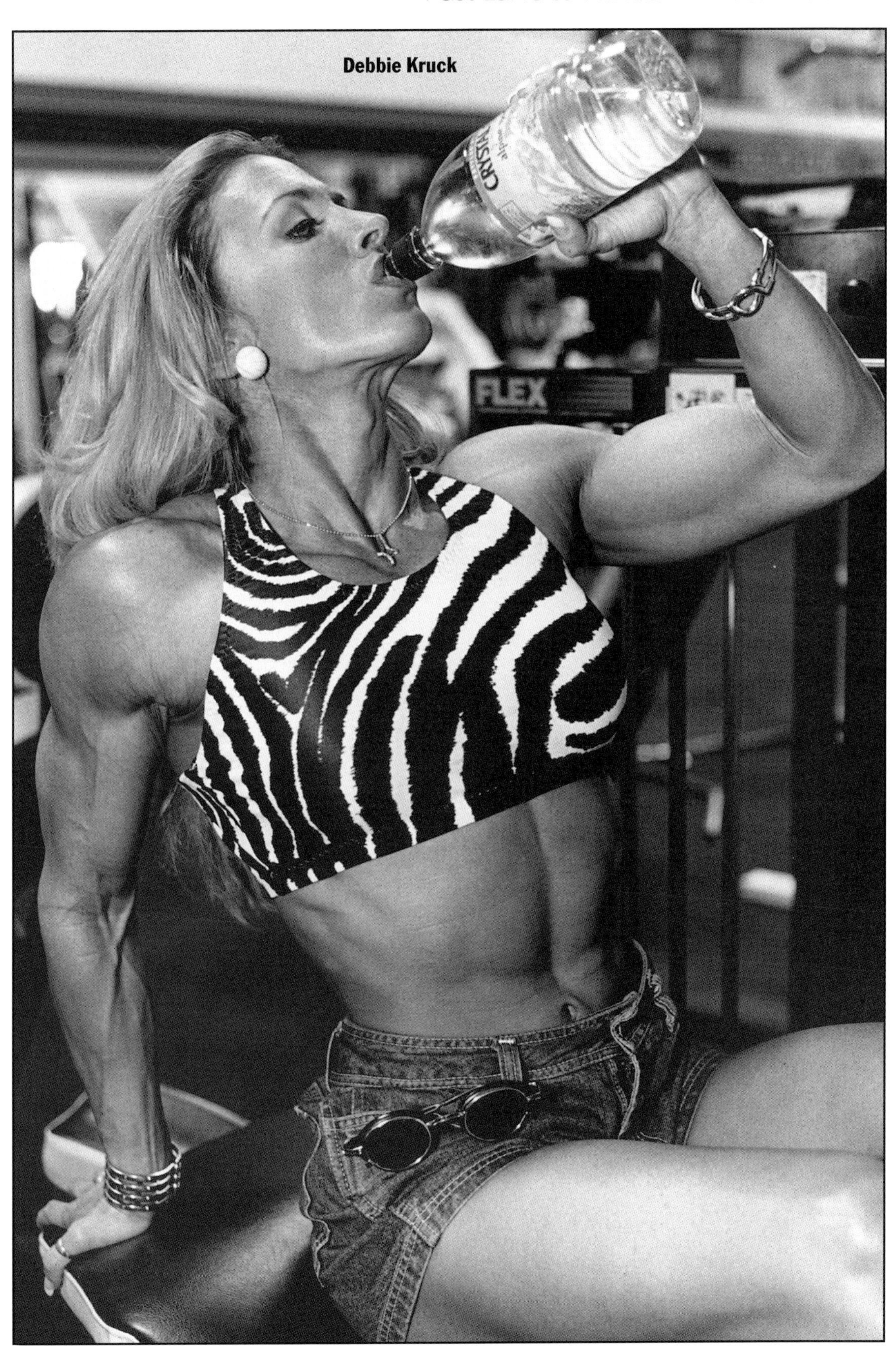

Debbie Kruck

Contibuting Photographers
Jim Amentler, Alex Ardenti, Reg Bradford,
Richard Finnegan, Irvin Gelb, Robert Kennedy,
J.M. Manion, Jason Mathas, Rick Schaff,
Randi Leigh Sidman, Rob Sims, Rafael Tongol